D1566102

keep
yourself
thin

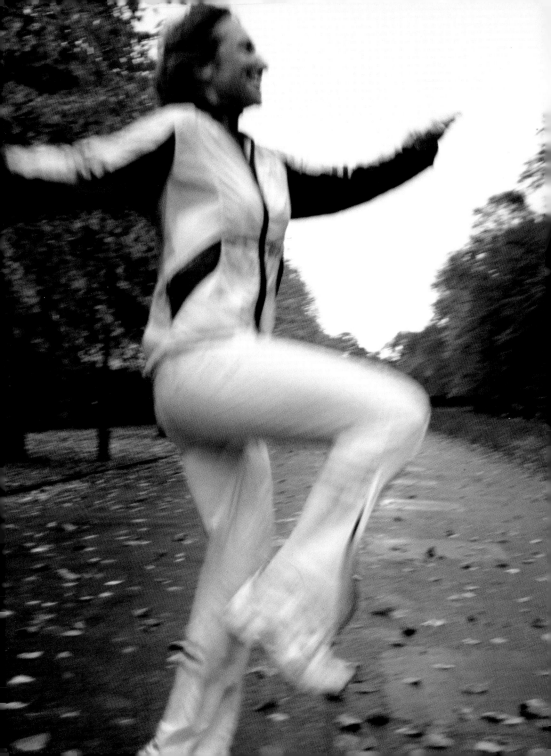

joanna hall

AFTER
THE DIET,
THE KEY TO
LONG-TERM
SUCCESS

keep
yourself
thin

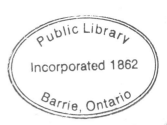

First published in Great Britain in 2008 by Kyle Cathie Limited
Kyle Cathie Limited
122 Arlington Road, London NW1 7HP
www.kylecathie.com
The material in this book comes from Joanna Hall's *The Weight-Loss Bible*

10 9 8 7 6 5 4 3 2 1

ISBN 978-1-85626-837-0

Project editor Vicki Murrell
Designer Abby Franklin
Photographer Dan Welldon
Production Sha Huxtable

A CIP record for this title is available from the British Library.

Printed by TWP, Singapore

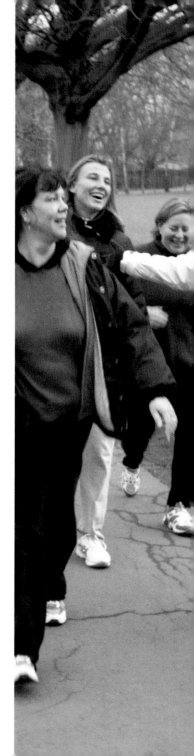

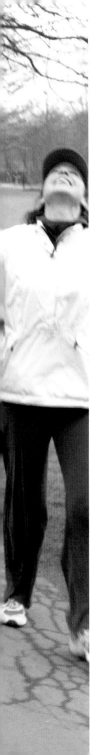

Contents

Introduction   6

1 So let's get to know you   8
- 7 steps to raise self-esteem ▪ motivation
- setting your goals ▪ barrier bashing

2 Where are you now?   26
- a question of size ▪ systems of measurement
- what shape are you? ▪ life journey of a body
- action plans

3 Making it happen   56
- navigating your day ▪ barrier bashing
- treat yourself

4 Your children's weight   84
- why are children gaining weight?
- the importance of exercise

5 Questions & Answers   102

Resources   110
Index   112

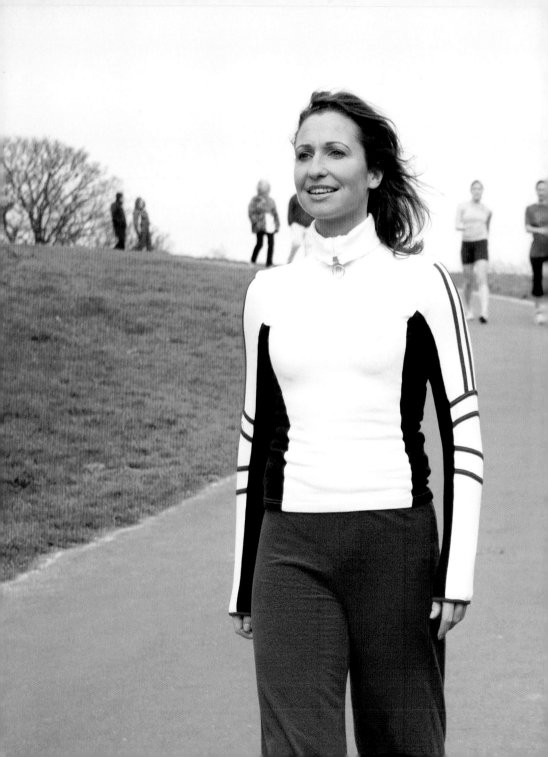

Introduction

After 15 years running weight-management programmes and helping real people who live real lives get real results, I'm familiar with the challenges of weight reduction: we may all wish for the perfect time to start a weight-loss and better-body campaign, but the fact is, life will always have little hiccups and dramas to throw us off our good intentions. Therefore, in this book, I want to excite you about what you can achieve, empower you with the skills to cope with the challenges and show you what can really work for you – helping you not just to get the weight off but also to keep it off and, most important of all, to feel good about yourself.

Weight loss is a journey and, as with any journey, there'll be high points and low points; there'll also be barriers blocking your path, but there are ways you can bash them down, as you'll see. You'll find loads of plans, ideas and practical tips to stop you feeling frustrated and start feeling successful. Before long, you'll realise you've become much more empowered; you'll have faith in your actions, and feel excited about what you can achieve. I've written this book for you to enjoy success, maintain your success, and feel confident in the knowledge that you've adopted a healthier way of living that won't just work for you today, but tomorrow as well, whatever your age or stage of life.

But for sustained weight loss, you need to ask yourself some basic questions first! You are the most important person on this journey, and you come first – not your partner, not your boss. So before you start, you need to know exactly who it is you are dealing with. Spending some time getting to know yourself a little better is an essential step, as the answers to the questions you ask yourself will have a direct effect on how you are able to keep the weight off and not let all your hard work go to waste. Remember this is about you and your life – and how you can do this for you. If this approach makes you feel guilty, just think: if you feel better about yourself, the other people around you will benefit too.

Be active

Joanna

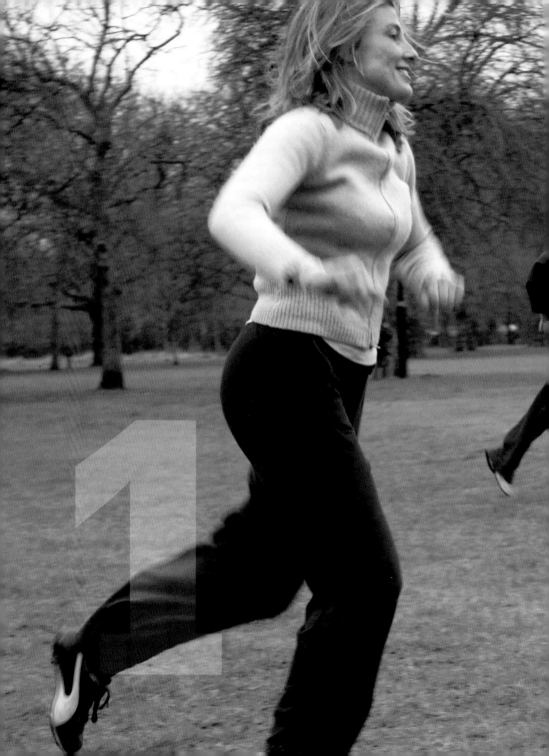

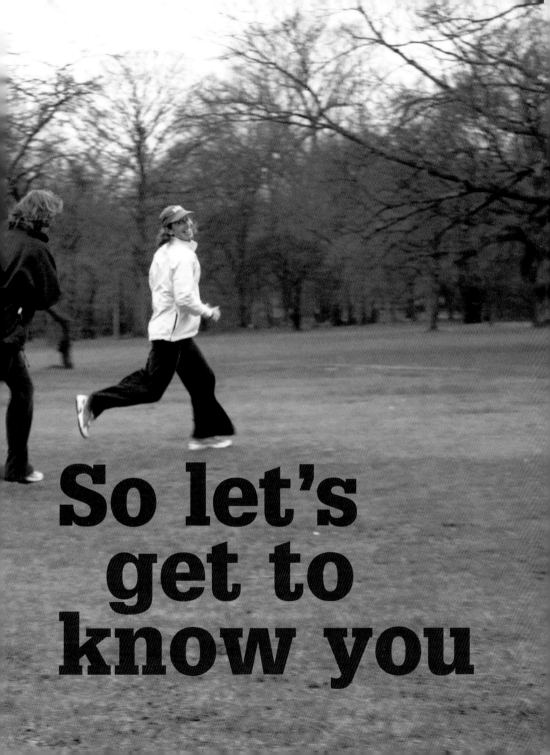

So let's get to know you

Where are you now and where are you going?

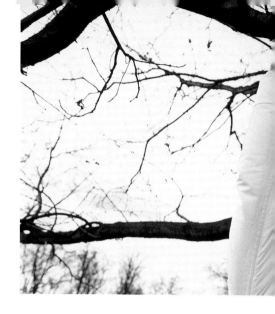

Sometimes the effort we think we have to make in order to get results appears just a little too daunting, and we can end up so terrified by the idea that we become less active than before. So let's stop right there!

Perhaps you think you have a pretty good idea of who you are, but the journey we are going on will require you to get to know yourself in quite a different way, almost as if you are another person; in fact, you will need to develop a 'relationship' with yourself. This involves taking a step back, and then a long, hard look at how your brain and your body work.

You need to think about:
- how your weight has changed over the years
- what exercise you like or don't like to do
- what foods you like to eat
- why you like to eat
- when you eat fattening foods.

How many times have you beaten yourself up for eating a whole packet of biscuits? Or got really frustrated with yourself when you decided to go out with your friends instead of going to the gym – despite promising yourself you would do both? How often have you opted for the less healthy choice on the restaurant menu when you knew quite well what would be better for you? Getting cross with yourself, or despairing at your lack of willpower, will do little for your self-esteem, and can directly undermine your efforts.

However, if you can see your own thought processes objectively – in effect, develop a relationship with your brain – you'll come to understand how it works. You'll see when it is hampering your

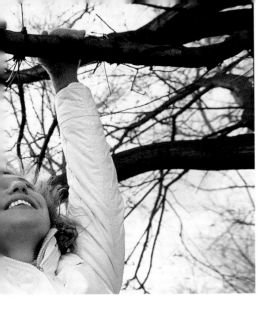

efforts and, in time, this will give you more confidence, as you will be able to get the better of your negative thoughts. You'll come to trust yourself, and have faith in your abilities.

THE BOTTOM LINE

The way you think about yourself can have just as powerful a role as the way you eat and the way you move your body. You need to train your brain and your body to work together in your fight against the flab. Like any relationship worth sustaining, the connection between your brain and body needs nurturing to remain strong. Don't neglect it.

Acknowledge that sadness, fear and other negative emotions can be turned around so that they help you learn and heal, celebrate and get the most out of life.

CHANGE YOUR TEMPLATE OF FAILURE TO A TEMPLATE OF SUCCESS

The whole ethos of this book is about you achieving success, whatever may be happening in your life to make it difficult. A key to this is feeling confident – about yourself, and about the journey we're taking together – providing a firm foundation for your Template of Success. Don't worry; this can't miraculously happen overnight. But have faith in yourself, and in what we are doing, and it will strengthen your efforts. Work at it step by step, safe in the knowledge that everything is in place to support you. Let's start off by reinforcing some vital points. First of all, putting yourself first.

7 steps
to raise your
self-esteem

This section takes you through the strategies that will help you understand the importance of engaging not just your body but also your brain in your weight loss efforts. Each step builds upon the next, like the skin of an onion, taking you closer to the next layer and leading you towards your goal of creating a solid, stronger and more motivated whole.

Because each strategy builds the foundation for the next, you will need to go through each one methodically, and feel happy with it in order to progress. You may find some of the steps easier than others, but each is an important aspect to keeping off the weight you have lost.

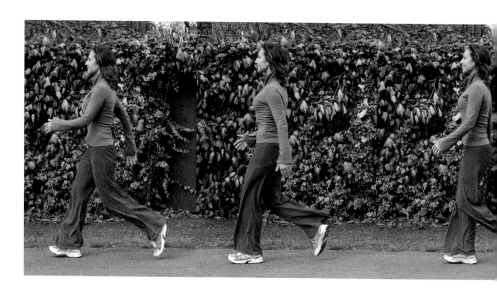

This section isn't just something you'll read through once and forget about. As you go through life, there will be times when your weight fluctuates and your resolve falters, and you need to get back on track. You may well find that you need to revisit this section, because what was originally an easy strategy to master could, at a different time of your life, become more significant and challenging. It's not a bad idea to reaffirm your worth once a year by looking at the answers you gave to each of the seven exercises on the following pages when you last did them, and evaluating how much progress you have made in the intervening time. Why not dedicate a special self-esteem notebook for this purpose?

GETTING RID OF NEGATIVITY

Feeling guilty or angry with yourself about minor day-to-day events is one thing, but if your whole life is dominated by negative emotions relating to something that has happened in the past, you may need the help of a counsellor or therapist to resolve the issues (contact the British Association of Counselling and Psychotherapy, www.bacp.co.uk). Remember: whatever you did then, and whatever you do now, you were, and are, doing the best you can in the circumstances.

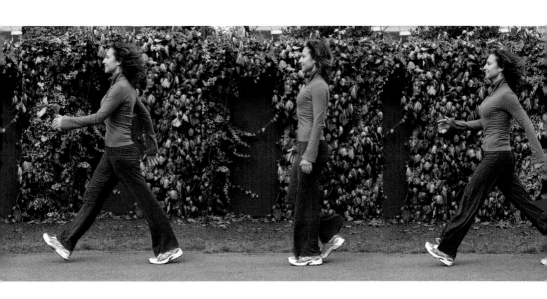

1. ACKNOWLEDGE YOUR ACHIEVEMENTS

What you need to do: Acknowledge the great things you have accomplished in your life. Take credit for your accomplishments and don't belittle them by dismissing them as merely 'OK' or 'not bad'– use big, positive, bold words that truly reflect your achievements. Shout it out!

The logic: Too many of us down-play our triumphs, sometimes so others can feel more secure. At school we are taught to be modest, with the 'good' pupils promoting the others around them, never themselves. This modesty can actually undermine and sabotage confidence because as we progress through our lives, fewer and fewer of us receive compliments or positive feedback on our performance. If you can't even acknowledge, let alone shout about, your own accomplishments, they go unnoticed by the most important person – YOU. And remember: if you don't value what you do, it's a cue for others to do the same.

2. LIST YOUR SUCCESSES

What you need to do: Make a list of all the things you decided you wanted to do in your life and then managed to accomplish. Include everything you can think of, from putting up shelves to passing your driving test to changing your own flat tyre or getting a promotion at work. You'll probably surprise yourself with how much you have already achieved, and this will spur you on.

The logic: The action of recalling events or situations in which you have met a challenge builds your confidence: you have the ability to translate your thinking and saying into action.

3. REVISIT PAST ACTS OF BRAVERY

What you need to do: If you are feeling demoralised or unable to face a situation for fear of rejection or failure, then recounting acts of bravery at other times or in other areas of your life can remind you that you are capable of confronting difficulties. To trigger these memories, sketch out a time line spanning from kindergarten to adult life. Try to jot down ten courageous acts. If you cannot remember, ask a friend or older member of the family. It doesn't matter how small – maybe it was deciding to own up to something when you were little, or going to a party where you knew your ex would be with his new girlfriend. Beside each event, write down the outcome of the situation.

The logic: Revisiting the past and citing even the smallest of brave acts can remind you of your bravery. As we get older, our brain often forgets these small acts and instead we tend to focus on what we feel we have not been able to address and overcome. Even the most timid of people will have had fearless moments – the trick is to remind yourself.

4. STEP INTO THE TARDIS

What you need to do: Make a list of past situations that you were fearful of or worried about. Next, record how you dealt with the situation and decide whether you feel you handled it successfully or not. Finally, note how you think you could have improved the outcome by using a different approach or strategy.

The logic: Your attitude to weight management will involve a series of strategies and approaches to get the outcome you want. Looking at situations that have caused you hurt or problems in the past and how you have dealt with them requires you to assess your stategies. It also enables you to see that a desired outcome is not always immediate.

5. THINK CHALLENGE, NOT PROBLEM

What you need to do: It's that old chestnut – is your glass half full or half empty? Whether you believe it or not, start telling yourself right now that it is half full. The more often you say it, the more you will come to believe it. Without getting evangelical, this new outlook will energise you to get what you want.

The logic: How you view a situation can have a significant impact on how you deal with it. So stop looking at the difficulties life throws at you as 'problems', but instead see them as challenges that throw forward new ways for you to look at your situation and learn about yourself and others. Use these challenges as opportunities to deepen your resourcefulness and move closer towards your goals.

6. BE AN EARLY BIRD

What you need to do: Each day, aim to do the things you least want to do first. Leave the nice things until afterwards, like a child who leaves their favourite food on the plate till last. You will be able to deal with the things you would otherwise put off far more effectively, and your actions will empower you through other activities in your day.

The logic: This way, you no longer have something unpleasant hanging over you. Research shows also that we are better able to deal with challenging situations in the morning as levels of the stress hormones cortisol and adrenaline are naturally higher at this time. Make the most of your biochemicals!

7. FORGIVE YOURSELF

What you need to do: Start right now by saying sorry to yourself. Say sorry for the way you have given yourself a hard time over an issue in your life, no matter how big or small. Acknowledge why it happened and forgive yourself. Then move forward.

The logic: Everyone screws up sometimes, but the important thing is to acknowledge the error and move on. Negative emotions, such as depression, guilt and cynicism, were associated with higher abdominal fat distribution in a study at Pennsylvania State University because of their association with higher cortisol. Harbouring negative feelings won't help you achieve anything.

Putting yourself on a pedestal

Right – we are going to play a game. This game is about finding out where you figure on your list of priorities. You'll need a pen and a piece of paper.

Write the numbers 1 to 7 down the left-hand side of the piece of paper. Decide who is the most important person in your life and write the name beside the number 1. After that, who is the next most important person in your life? Write the name beside the number 2. Ask yourself this question seven times, and write down your answers by each number in order.

How do you score this game? If you get to six or seven strikes and you don't see your name on the list, you are done for! Why? Because if you are that low down your priority list, then your weight-loss attempts will fail. Your needs are not important enough for you to give them the time and energy they require. You do not value yourself enough.

Now ask yourself who is responsible for caring for all those other people who are more important than you. Chances are, it is you. Let's get one thing straight: if you feel low about yourself, making sensible eating and other lifestyle choices becomes harder, and your health suffers. And don't think that it is just you that's affected. You don't just give yourself a hard time but also possibly jeopardise the smooth running of your family, your home and the very people you care about.

There's one thing that we have to establish before we go any further... you are not going to succeed in your weight-loss journey unless your motivation is strong, and the best, truest motivation is the one that benefits you and you alone. Determining your true motivation is the next step.

TAKE WHAT YOU NEED

Many people complain that they do not have enough time to eat healthily, take regular exercise and manage stress, but the issue is not always about making time. It is about taking time. Taking time is only possible when you feel you are worthy of it. Being happy to take time involves raising yourself a few rungs up the ladder. Even if you are not at the top of the list, getting higher is important. Taking time out is not about being selfish, it's about self-care.

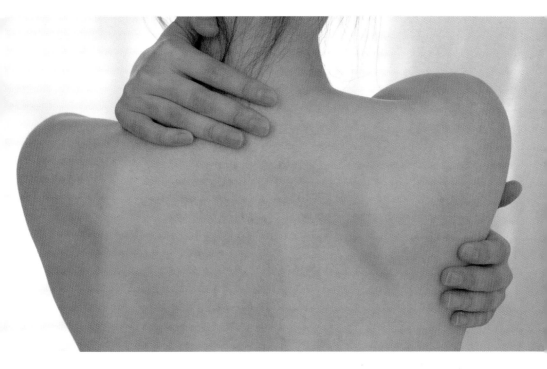

GET NAKED

Develop a relationship with your cells. Go on – take your clothes off right now and stand in front of a full-length mirror. YES, right now. Give yourself a good long hard look and say: 'If I want to see a change in my body shape [a leaner body, slimmer thighs or whatever your goals may be], I need to develop a relationship with my body and specifically a relationship with my cells.'

Your cells are tiny microscopic units in your body that carry out your everyday needs, and are responsible for using your body's energy effectively and the food you eat efficiently. Developing a good relationship with your cells is like a friendship; if you treat them well then they repay your kindness. If, on the other hand, you go on erratic starvation diets and suddenly start exercising excessively, your cells will be confused and will not know how to respond. The net result will be that your energy will flag and your weight-loss efforts start to flounder, despite what you perceive as putting in masses of hard work. So be kind to your cells – they want to help you.

So now you know what shape you're in and what you're up against – we've come a long way already. With both your brain and your body working together, we're ready to go on to the next stage, and find out what you need to do.

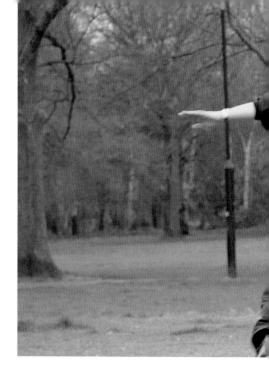

The G spot motivation

Open any women's magazine and you'll be reminded that finding your G spot heightens your enjoyment of sex. It's something that both you and your partner will want to do, since once you enjoy something, you start to want more.

If you want to keep the weight off, you need to find your G spot for weight loss. What is your long-term motivation to keep your size down? For many, finding your true G spot for weight loss, as in sex, can be difficult. And it's no good having some vague idea and faking it. In the end it'll give you no satisfaction at all.

What is your current motivation? It may be to look good in a bikini on a summer holiday with your best friend, for a special occasion or perhaps even your wedding day. These are short-lived – you haven't quite got there. If you really want

to stay slim, you have to come up with something that will give you lasting pleasure, and keep those inches off for life.

Ask yourself what you really want to achieve with your weight loss. What is it about being slimmer that you think will make you ultimately happier, ultimately more fulfilled? Maybe it's social confidence, or perhaps the freedom to wear what you want, or the thought of enjoying a good night's sleep. Or perhaps feeling fitter and having the freedom and energy to do more will give you lasting satisfaction? Think about it.

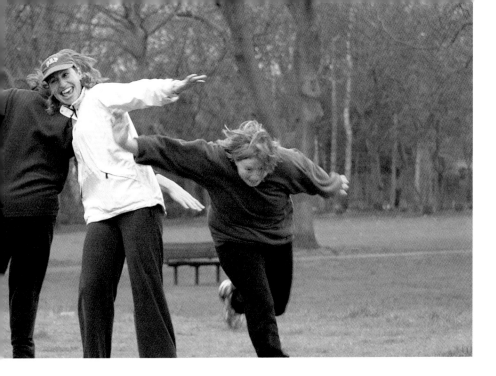

RECALL OTHER TIMES WHEN YOU WERE MOTIVATED

What you need to do: Think back to an event or period when you were truly driven to do something – perhaps it was to get through your professional qualifications, recover from an operation, or plan a surprise party for someone. Whatever it was, you were strongly motivated to make it happen.

The logic: Realise that if you were strong enough to have the motivation to accomplish those achievements, then you have the ability to apply the same strength to losing weight. Tap into that motivational strength and you can use it to help you reach your goal.

START TO HEAL YOURSELF

What you need to do: This is a simple game to help you identify how large your G spot motivation is. Make two lists: in the first, make a note of all your harmful lifestyle habits, and in the second, think of a healing substitute. Now decide which harmful habits you are prepared to replace with the things that are ultimately going to get you what you want. Next, ask yourself how long you are prepared to do this for – is it a day, a week, a fortnight, a month, or longer?

The logic: If you're only prepared to do this for a short period, you'll never be really satisfied with the result, and will constantly yo-yo between guilt and virtue. Otherwise, wow! You'll never look back.

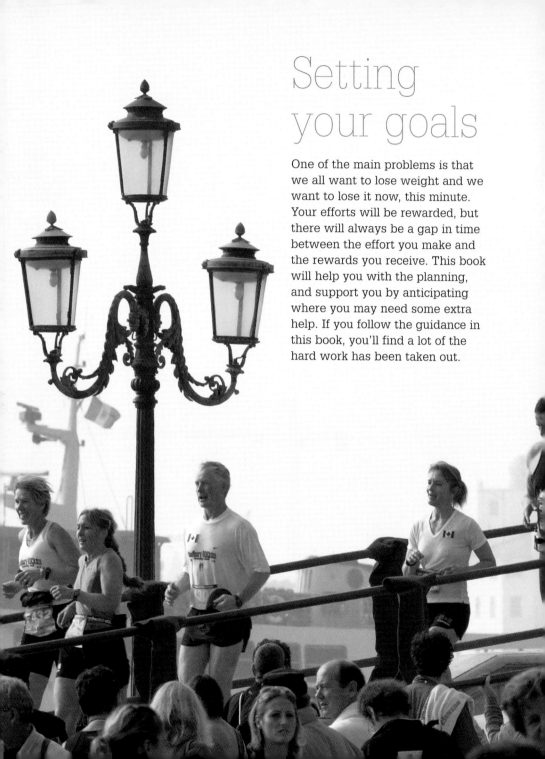

Setting your goals

One of the main problems is that we all want to lose weight and we want to lose it now, this minute. Your efforts will be rewarded, but there will always be a gap in time between the effort you make and the rewards you receive. This book will help you with the planning, and support you by anticipating where you may need some extra help. If you follow the guidance in this book, you'll find a lot of the hard work has been taken out.

The essential point with goal setting is to make sure your target is realistic and achievable. A lot has been written about goal setting and weight loss and with good reason, because so many difficulties can arise if your goal is unachievable within the time set. Realistic weight loss is around 1kg (2^1/$_4$lbs) a week – although this will depend on your dieting history, the consistency of your effort and your own metabolism. Your rate of change will vary but, as a rule of thumb, it is not unrealistic to be able to drop a clothes size in four weeks. Aiming for a weight loss of 1kg a week is sensible; however, bear in mind the fact that the rate at which you lose it may not be consistent.

Think about this: Remember your weight five years ago – and imagine a straight line from there to here, the present moment. Logically, then, you can extend that line and see where you'll be in five years' time if you continue with your current eating and exercise habits. If that place isn't where you want to be with your body, your health and your shape, then you need to address your thoughts, decisions and actions right now. The present is on the same straight line as the past and future, so if you want to change direction, act now. You can do this.

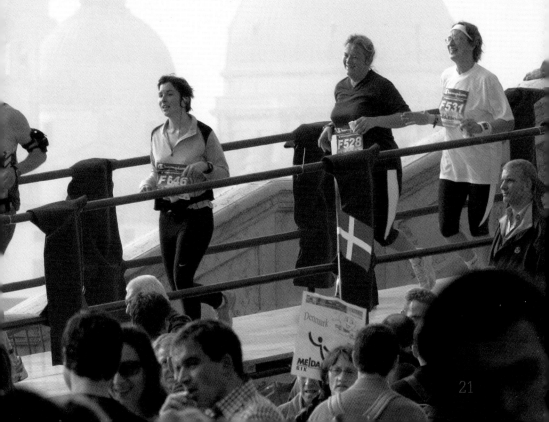

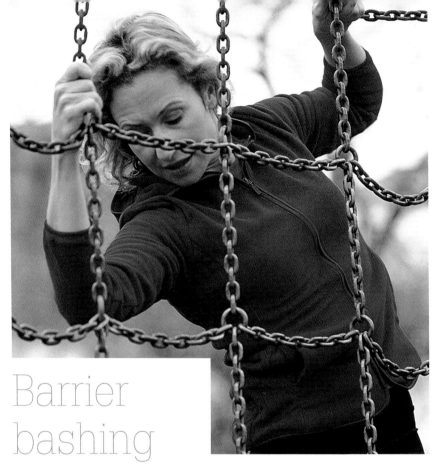

Barrier bashing

On your weight-loss journey you are going to come up against a whole host of barriers that can hinder your efforts. Many will be genuine challenges, possibly the same ones that have hindered your progress in the past. So deciding on a way to deal with them and bash them down will be part of your weight-loss tool kit. The logic concerning barriers is simple: when they are high, or perceived to be high, then confidence is low. Identifying your barriers in advance and learning how to bash them down will help keep you on track. In this book you'll come across several barriers, but you'll also find ways to help you become a great Barrier Basher! Remember: if you do not attempt to implement some of the action plans to break the barriers down, then your barrier still exists. Learning to bash down your barriers can help you to become an Inner Coach rather than an Inner Critic.

BARRIER: LACK OF TIME

Probably the most cited barrier. You don't need to have hours on end to take action, or put your normal life on hold to make weight loss work for you.

Bash it down: Exercise earlier in the day. Studies have shown that people who are new to exercise and choose to exercise first thing in the morning are 75 per cent more likely to still be exercising 12 months later. Schedule in exercise blocks at the start of each week and write reminders everywhere – on your computer screen, diary, mobile phone and post-it notes – to let you know when you should be exercising. Think shorter exercise bouts, not longer! Research has shown that people who take shorter exercise bouts end up completing more than those whose exercise bouts were longer (International Journal of Obesity, 1995). Seek out ways to exercise at home. People tend to stick with home-based exercises more than facility-based exercise sessions (Perri et al., 1997).

BARRIER: TOO MUCH EFFORT

Many people perceive exercise as a skill, requiring great physical co-ordination or an aptitude for sport – but this needn't be the case.

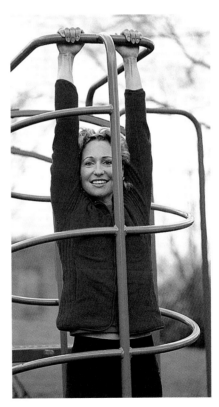

Bash it down: Seek out ways to exercise at home. For example, use home exercise DVDs, or try walking routes of differing lengths near your home. Stop looking at exercise purely as a way of getting hot and sweaty, or as something that has to be done in exercise kit. Building up lifestyle activity to top up your structured exercise can help change your traditional perceptions about exercise.

BARRIER: LACK OF SUPPORT

Social support is very important, whether it is from a partner, friend or support group. There will be people, however, who discourage your new healthy habits.

Bash it down: Seek out and identify who will be the supporters and saboteurs. Studies with recovering heart disease patients reveal that men had an 80 per cent adherence rate to their exercise programme when supported by their spouse compared to 40 per cent when their spouse had a neutral attitude.

Find exercise partners who will be powerful motivational supporters. Find people who can help make it easier to build exercise into your life. For example, if your partner or friend agrees to pick up the children three days a week, you can use that time to exercise. Explaining to others the importance to you of following your exercise and eating programme may help them be more supportive.

BARRIER: LACK OF SELF-ESTEEM

Building self-confidence in yourself right now is crucial. Don't wait for your self-confidence to suddenly appear once you have lost weight. Invest in it now.

Bash it down: Teach yourself small successes. Take 120 micro-bouts of 15 seconds' exercise throughout the day and you've done 30 minutes of exercise without even realising it. Congratulate yourself with post-it reminders each time you complete your actions. Regularly re-visit the steps to self-esteem on pages 12–15.

BARRIER: LACK OF KNOWLEDGE

You want to lose weight but you don't know where to start, what plan to follow, what exercise to do or what food to eat. A lack of knowledge can be just as confusing as having too much information and not knowing where to start.

Bash it down: Make a commitment to learning about how your body works and the impact your actions, however small, can have. Invest in yourself and enrol on a course with a qualified personal trainer or weight-management support group, or join my online walk off weight club (www.walkactive.co.uk) – we provide lots of support and there is an incredible choice of events to attend.

Be specific about what you want to achieve, so your plan can be as appropriate as possible.

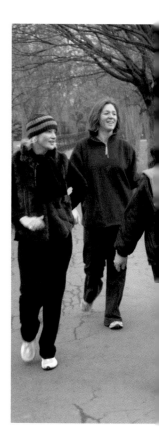

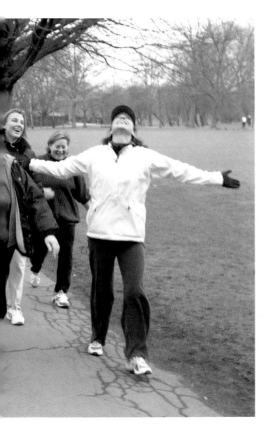

BARRIER: TOO MANY OBSTACLES

Hindrances such as not being near a health club or having to work late, the menstrual cycle or a weekend away with friends can all be obstacles that act as a barrier.

Bash it down: Honestly identify your behaviour chains. These are the chains of events that can stop you from exercising or eating sensibly. For example, you may have planned to go to the gym after work but you ended up not going because your boss shoved a report under your nose as you were walking out the door and said he wanted it ready for first thing the following morning. You may blame your lack of gym attendance on the actions of your boss, but in actual fact, the real reason could be because you overslept, which put pressure on your day from the start. If you plan the next day before you go to bed, it can make a big difference to what you realistically achieve.

WHAT IS SUCCESS?

Measuring your success plays a very important part in sustaining your weight-loss motivation. But what constitutes success? Success may primarily mean victory on the scales, but your success will also be reflected in a far wider range of changes than this – and learning about them now will be helpful when your weight loss slows down or even stays the same for a while, despite your continued efforts. (This is quite normal; it should be something you're prepared for.)

Positive side-effects of weight loss success will include having more energy, sleeping better, reducing high blood pressure or blood cholesterol, dropping belt buckle-holes, increased confidence, noticing a more radiant complexion and a spring in your step, and not feeling short of breath as you walk up the stairs... The list is endless, so note down your own particular successes. There will be far more than just the decreasing measurements on your bathroom scales.

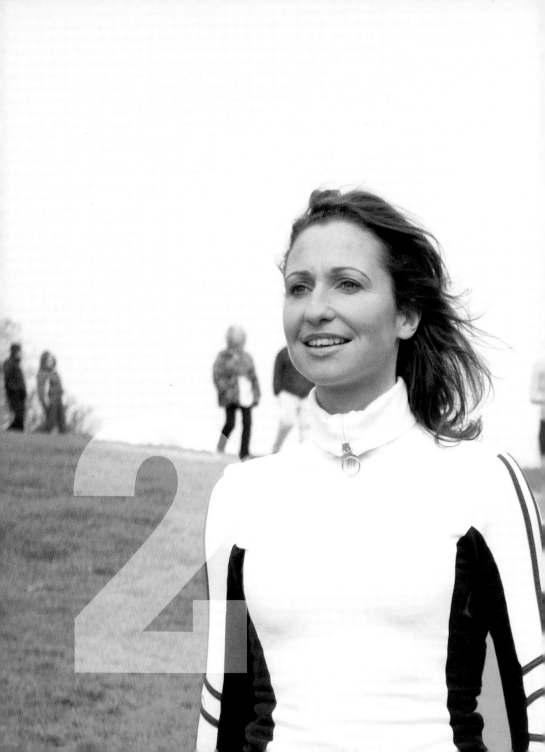

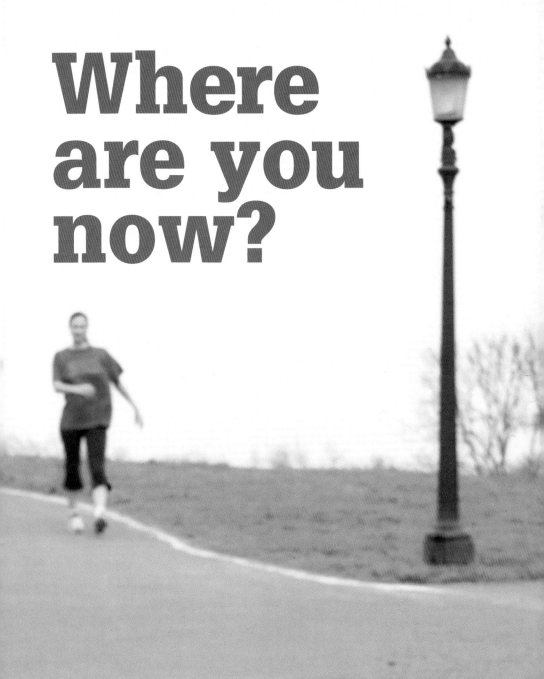

Where are you now?

Facts and figures

You have got to know yourself a little better, and you are all ready to go. But do you know the point you're starting from? What kind of shape is your body in at the moment? This chapter is all about finding out.

DO I REALLY NEED TO KNOW?

Yes. Establishing what shape you're in now will give you a baseline that you can use as your starting point. Studies have shown conclusively that the more accountable weight-loss participants are, the more successful their outcome. So self-monitoring is a crucial part.

WHAT DO I MEASURE?

I would strongly encourage you to measure both your body shape and your body composition, and there is a number of ways you can do this. Some methods are simpler than others, so choose the one that you feel best able to work with. Many have different definitions and thresholds of obesity, which can often lead to confusion when you are trying to establish whether or not you fall within a healthy range.

Your body is made up of lean muscle tissue and adipose (fat) tissue around a skeleton, which forms a framework for your body shape. From a health perspective, the most significant factor is the amount of adipose tissue you have. Our bodies hold adipose fat internally around delicate organs such as the liver, kidneys and heart and, more visibly, it is also stored under the surface of the skin and on top of the muscles, which lie over our skeletal framework. Some adipose tissue is also stored inside our muscles. If you are putting on weight, this will be most apparent in the fat deposits of the adipose tissue under the skin; however, additional fat will also be stored around our delicate organs and in our muscles, posing some serious health risks.

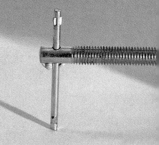

HOW OFTEN SHOULD I MEASURE?

This is up to you, and partly depends upon what suits you and what will most effectively support you and keep you on track on your weight-loss journey. As a rule, I encourage my clients to use one simple form of measurement once a week and another more comprehensive system once a month. For example, weigh yourself once a week and take a set of body circumference measurements on the first day of each month. And ladies, remember: a woman can put on up to 2kg (4lb) at the time of her period just through fluid retention.

WHEN SHOULD I MEASURE?

Again this is up to you, but in my experience the start of the week is the best time. This helps prevent you from splurging during your leisure time at the weekend and also serves to focus you for the week ahead. Whether you measure first thing in the morning or later in the day will make no difference to your overall weight-loss progression – the important thing is to measure at the same time each time, either without clothes or wearing the same garments. Some measurements take into account your body's water content, so time of day may be specific to them. Measuring at the same time will give you a proper baseline to keep returning to.

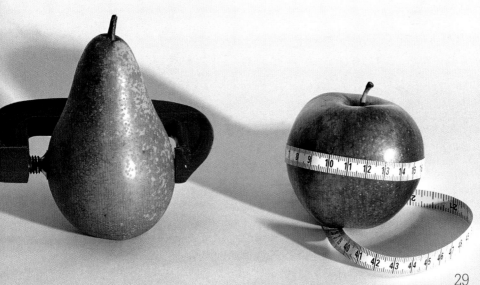

Systems of measurements

There is a wide variety of systems available, each of them measuring a different aspect of body fat and with varying degrees of accuracy. This helps to explain why somebody may be classified as having a healthy weight according to one system but overweight according to another. Obviously this can prove confusing, so although you may be interested to see how you compare using all the methods of measurement, I suggest that you select just one or two, and be consistent with your measuring.

THE BATHROOM SCALES

What they do? Show you how much you weigh.

The healthy range It is difficult to give healthy range targets, although a 5–10 per cent decrease in excess weight can lead to a significantly reduced risk of chronic disease and disability. Use scales in conjunction with your BMI or waist circumference to give you a healthy range to work towards.

The drawbacks Since they account for the weight of your muscle, fat and skeletal system as a whole they do not tell you the amount of body fat you have or its distribution.

The benefits One of the easiest measures to take (and of course, the most widely used). Just be brave and stand on a set of good, calibrated scales.

BODY MASS INDEX (BMI)

What it does BMI measures your weight in relation to your height. To establish your BMI, measure your height in metres and your weight in kilograms, and then divide your weight by your height squared:

$$W \div H^2 = BMI$$

For example, you weigh 63kg (10 stone) and are 1.70m (5ft 7in) tall.
  1.70 x 1.70 = 2.89
  63 ÷ 2.89 = 21.79

The healthy range A normal BMI should fall between 18.5 and 24.9. Anything between 24.9 and 29.9 is considered overweight and above that qualifies as obese. Once you know your weight and height you can get your BMI automatically calculated at www.joannahall.com.

The drawbacks The BMI does not distinguish between fat and muscle, nor does it take into account where your body fat is distributed. This is important because it is not just the amount or the composition of excess weight that affects health, but its regional distribution – where the extra fat is stored within the body. It's also not a good measure of progress as you get fitter, since increased muscle mass may actually make you heavier, although you will be substantially leaner and trimmer and your clothes should fit better.

The benefits The BMI is a widely used measurement of obesity. Many GPs and medical establishments talk about BMI, so knowing your BMI score is useful.

WAIST CIRCUMFERENCE

What it does? Measures round your middle (a normal tape measure will do).

The healthy range It has been suggested that if waist circumference rises above 90cm (35^1/$_2$in) in men and above 80cm (31^1/$_2$in) in women, the risk of metabolic complications is increased. Weight reduction is strongly advised if waist circumference is more than 102cm (40in) in men and 88cm (35in) in women, as this represents a significantly increased medical risk.

The drawbacks Reduction in waist circumference may take some time to materialise, so it's advisable to use this method in conjunction with another body measurement that may be more sensitive to changes, such as weight. It has been recommended that sex-specific waist circumference cut-off points need to be developed for different populations because people from different ethnic backgrounds vary in their level of risk for diseases such as coronary heart disease and Type 2 diabetes (World Health Organisation, 2000).

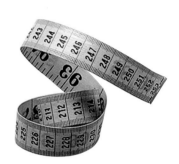

The benefits Very easy to do. Recent evidence suggests that waist circumference on its own may prove very useful. It correlates closely with BMI and WHR (see below) and is a good index of intra-abdominal fat mass and total body fat.

WAIST-TO-HIP RATIO (WHR)

What it does? Identifies patients with abdominal fat accumulation. It is a recognised clinical method by which the waist is measured at the narrowest point and the hips are measured at the widest point. The waist measurement is then divided by the hip measurement.

The healthy range A high WHR is defined as above 1.0 in men and above 0.85 in women. A healthy range is below these two values.

The drawbacks Like waist circumference, WHR only identifies the distribution of your abdominal fat, so it's wise to use it in conjunction with another, more sensitive measure.

The benefits Like waist circumference, it's easy to do, using a simple tape measure and can be particularly interesting to monitor as we get older.

PERCENTAGE BODY FAT

What it does? Calculates the amount of fat your body contains in relation to your muscle mass.

The healthy range This depends on your age. For adults between 18 and 40, the healthy ranges are 18–26 per cent for men and 24–34 per cent for women.

The drawbacks A number of methods can be used to gauge percentage body fat, some more accurate than others. Underwater weighing is the most exact, although this is expensive and not widely available. More convenient methods include using hand-held callipers to take measurements at three to six sites on the body and then feeding these figures into a regression equation. Simpler still, you can stand on a set of special scales using a non-invasive technique called bioelectrical impedence. The scales can be used in your home, whereas the calliper method needs to be administered by a trained professional.

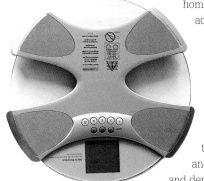

The benefits If you know your weight and your body fat percentage you can easily work out the weight of your fat and muscle, known as fat free mass and lean muscle mass respectively. Specially made scales available to measure children's body fat can be useful to avoid embarrassment in a clinical setting and are available from most large chemists and department stores.

KEEP IT SIMPLE

If you're still not sure which measuring system to use, my advice would be to keep it simple. Monitor your weight and either your waist measurement and/or girth measurements. And if even this feels unmanageable, I always think the old blue jeans measure – although not scientifically sound – can in many ways be the most personally powerful. Dig out that favourite piece of clothing that you can't fit into any more, and use that as your monthly reference point.

GIRTH MEASUREMENTS

What it does Measures body circumference at specific points (with a tape measure):

Chest: across the nipple line

Waist: around the narrowest part of your midriff

Navel: around the midriff, directly over the bellybutton

Hips: across the top of the buttock cheeks. This may not necessarily be the widest part of your hips.

Thighs: 20cm (8in) up from top of your kneecaps, standing with your feet together. (You will need some help when taking this measurement.)

The healthy range Except for the waist circumference measurement guidelines on page 31, there are no standard recognised reference ranges.

The drawbacks You may need some help to check that you are positioning the tape correctly.

The benefits Simple and cheap to do. Measuring at various sites can be more motivating, as different hormone distribution and concentration in different parts of the body will mean your body may change shape more in one part than another. Remember: any scrap of change is encouraging!

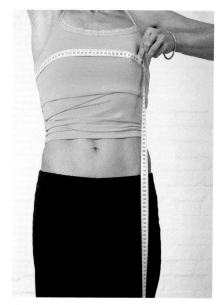

Chest

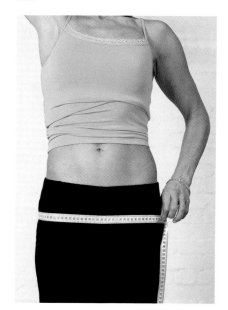

Hips

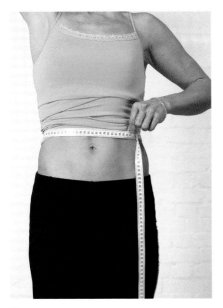

Waist

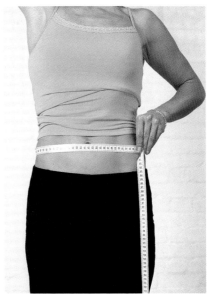

Navel

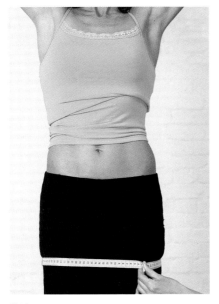

Thighs

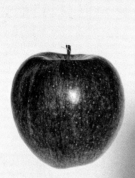
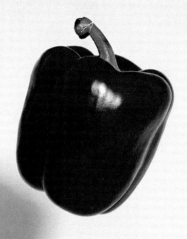

Body shape

We have become so used to seeing incredible celebrity body transformations on television and in magazines that we seem to expect the same level of transformation from our own body. In reality, however, most of us don't have the sort of money it takes – or the luxury of air-brushing. It is possible to improve our figures but exactly how much can we change the body shape Mother Nature dealt us?

Our fundamental body shape – skeletal frame, muscle, body fat and distribution of certain hormones – is determined by our genes. According to geneticist Claude Bouchaud, our genes and the hormones we produce during puberty can determine our body shape by as much as 70 per cent... so that leaves about 30 per cent that can be redefined, moulded and determined by exercise and what we eat.

As we get older our bodies naturally lose muscle, but muscle tone can be improved and muscle size can be increased with appropriate exercise. Body fat is directly determined by energy balance – consuming too many calories and not expending them increases body fat, while expending more calories than are consumed encourages body fat reduction. But unless we undergo significant cosmetic surgery, which is a very bad idea, our basic body shape – whether we're 'big-boned' or 'petite' – is pretty fixed.

We generally fall into four broad body shapes. I've categorised them as: pear, red pepper, carrot and apple.

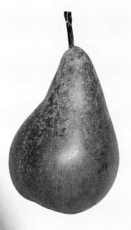
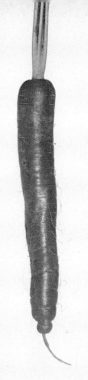

WHAT SHAPE ARE YOU?

You are more pear if:
- your hips are wider than your shoulders
- you have a smaller upper body frame
- your top half is 1 to 2 dress sizes smaller than your lower half.

You are more red pepper if:
- you have an ample bottom and bust with a defined waist
- you are a classic hourglass shape
- you are prone to gaining weight and storing body fat on arms and legs.

You are more carrot if:
- you have broadish shoulders with slimmer hips
- you have a smallish bottom and bust
- you tend not to hold excess fat around your midriff
- your waistline is not clearly defined.

You are more apple if:
- you store body fat around your midriff rather than hips and thighs
- you are shorter in height
- you have a flattish bottom.

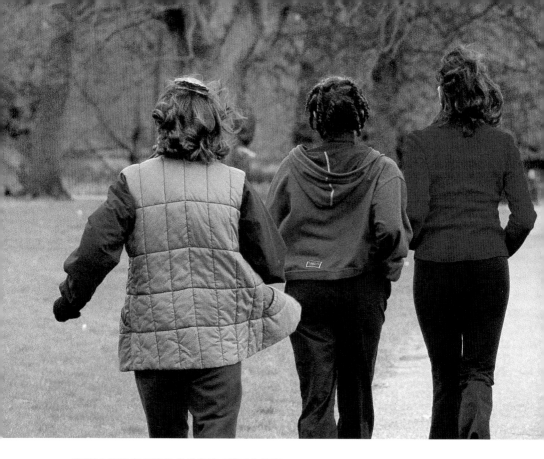

WHAT'S YOUR BODY FRAME?

Here is a quick way to identify the size of your body frame
– it's not scientifically proven but it will give you a rough idea.
Encircle your wrist with your thumb and middle finger.

If the middle finger overlaps your thumb, chances are you
are small-framed. If the middle finger and thumb touch, you
have a medium-sized body frame; and if the finger and thumb
do not touch you are more likely to have a larger frame.

Remember: for optimum health, all body types need a
balanced exercise programme involving a combination of
cardiovascular, resistance and flexibility work. But a particular
type may benefit from extra concentration on a specific
component. However, if in doubt, always think of your
cardiovascular work as your foundation.

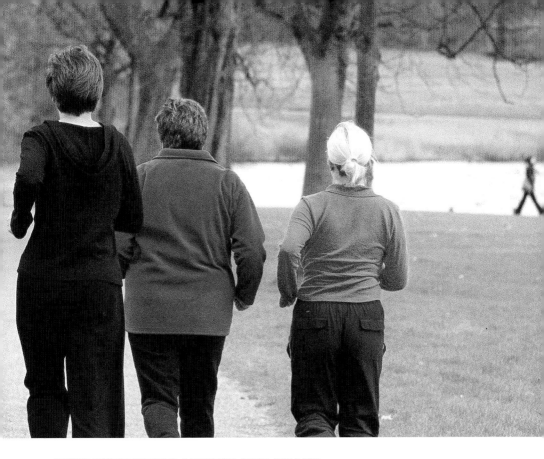

HOW HORMONES AFFECT OUR SHAPE

Some of us store more body fat on our hips and thighs while others tend to have long lean arms and legs but store more body fat around our midriffs. This distribution of fat is associated directly with two main hormones: lipoprotein lipase, or LPL, which encourages fat storage, and hormone-sensitive lipase, or HSL, which encourages fat to be distributed in the blood and then burnt off. The amount of LPL and HSL may vary from person to person and from one part of the body to another, directly affecting our shape.

- More LPL in the belly and less HSL in the lower hip area creates an apple-like shape, with more body fat distributed around the belly.
- More LPL in the hips and backs of the arms and less HSL in the upper body produces a pear-like shape.

This hormone distribution helps to explain why we still retain the same overall body shape when we lose weight.

The life journey of a body

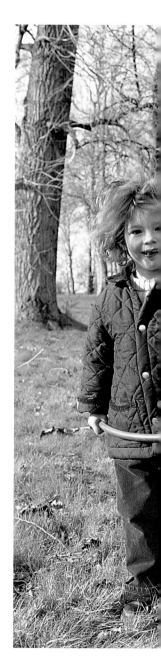

We may want to fit exercise into our schedules, but all too often our busy lifestyles prevent us from being as active as we would like. The weeks go by, the months add up and before we know it we have entered another decade. Just as our lives and lifestyles evolve, so too do our bodies change. What we need to do to keep ourselves fit and healthy in our youth is quite different from the requirements of a more mature body. But whatever your age or the challenges life throws at you, there are simple and effective opportunities to be active!

As your body accompanies you through life, certain biological changes will occur at particular stages that affect your shape and weight. A sedentary lifestyle and excessive calorie intake can compound their effects. Recognising these changes will help you develop an understanding of your body and how it responds on your weight-loss journey, and this will further enhance the relationship you have with your body and your brain.

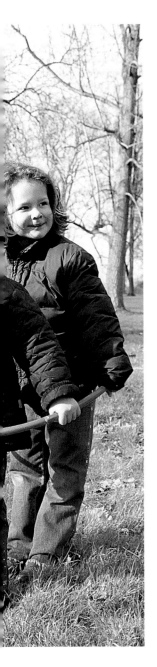

CHILDREN

Children have lower stroke volumes and higher heart rates than adults at all exercise intensities. In addition, both children and adolescents have higher maximum heart rates than adults, so methods for estimating maximum heart rates cannot be used for children or for adolescents until their late teens. Children and teenagers do not sweat as much as adults during exercise, as their sweat glands do not become fully effective until late in adolescence. This means that, when exercising in extreme cold or heat, they do not acclimatise so well and are more prone to heat exhaustion. Couple this with the fact that children do not have an effective thirst mechanism, and you have an age group which is susceptible to dehydration and heat exhaustion. Make sure your children drink plenty of fluids before, during and after exercise, as thirst may not be an accurate indicator of their requirements.

Ages 2–8

The focus of exercise in early childhood should be on the development of basic movement skills such as running, balancing, jumping and co-ordination. Exercise should centre around making movement fun. Yoga-style movements can be a great way for children to explore their bodies, incorporate all the movement skills and boost their physical self-confidence.

Ages 9–12

This is usually a time when children are becoming more aware of their bodies. Girls especially may be approaching puberty and this will heighten their self-awareness. In addition, work pressures at school will also be changing, more time will be spent on computers and less time allocated to physical movement. To avoid long periods of inactivity, schedule activity zones and technology-free zones with your family at the weekends. Encourage active pursuits such as roller-blading, football and skipping. Playful gizmos such as scooters and hoops can act as useful motivators to keep this age group interested in activity.

TEEN YEARS

During the teen years, focus on game-type activities which entertain as well as develop co-ordination. Older teens may be ready to concentrate on specific body areas and have exercise and physical-activity goals. They will be more aware of their bodies and may share adult concerns about weight loss and body shape. However, care needs to be taken to present a healthy message of moderate physical activity and not an obsession with body shape and size which can distort the teenager's perception of their body image. In addition, this age group may be more self-conscious and therefore more receptive to exercise if the sexes are separated.

Teenagers need cardiovascular conditioning to improve the health of heart and lungs and to stimulate bone plate loading (a process whereby the bone tissue is encouraged to become denser and stronger). Establishing the exercise habit as part of an active lifestyle is important, and parents need to look to themselves as pivotal role models in their children's attitude to activity. Group aerobics, team sports and yoga can all play a role in adolescent activity. School team sports such as basketball, football and hockey also provide an important opportunity for social interaction. However, if your children are naturally sporty, do encourage them to be active outside their sports.

Building in physical-activity habits that will stay with them for life is vitally important for long-term health. Studies have shown that being active in your younger years has no protective effect against heart disease and cancers if the physical activity is not maintained.

20s

Studies have shown that from the age of 25 our aerobic capacity decreases by 1–2 per cent each year. This means your heart and lungs have to work harder to complete everyday tasks, although you may not feel it until you have to overexert yourself – running for a bus, or dashing up several flights of stairs to answer the phone, for instance.

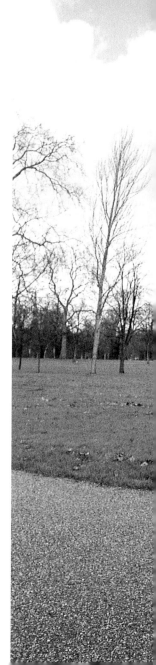

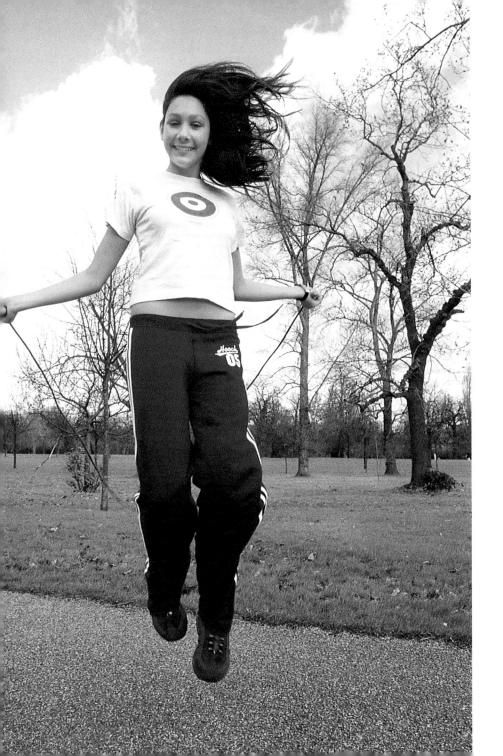

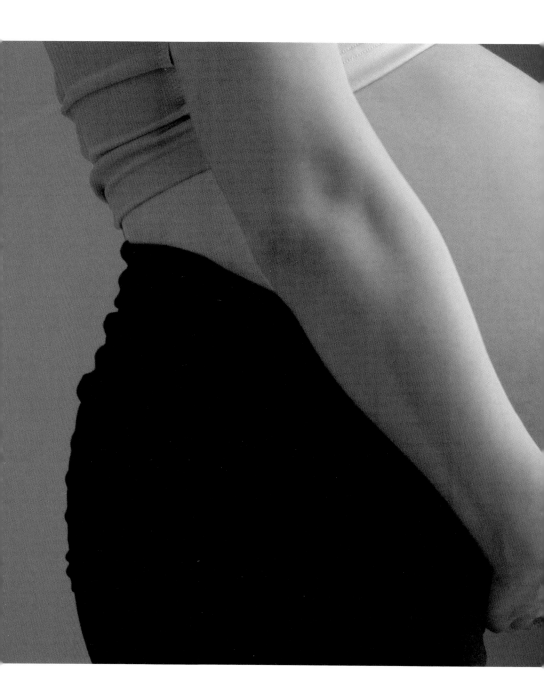

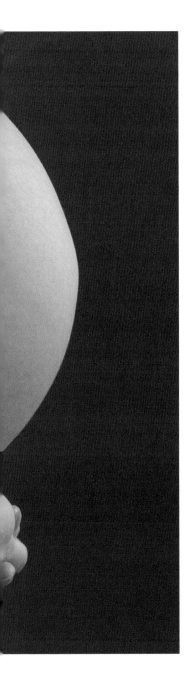

PREGNANCY

During pregnancy you gain weight and you need to gain weight. This results from a change in the concentration of hormones your body produces as well as from the growing baby and amniotic fluid inside. A woman of average build will put on around 10–12kg (20–24lb), mostly around the abdomen. If you find you are putting on much more weight than this (or not so much), then consult your doctor.

With sound advice, mums-to-be can continue (or even begin) to exercise during pregnancy. The American College of Obstetricians and Gynaecologists (ACOG) states that pregnant women can reap the health benefits associated with regular, mild to moderate exercise, providing that there are no complications with the pregnancy. Many women have found that regular exercise during pregnancy offsets the physiological changes the body is going through, as well as the psychological changes and inevitable weight gain.

How exercise can help

Exercise increases your cardiovascular stamina so that you can cope more easily with the demands of pregnancy. It can help to reduce minor related ailments such as varicose veins, constipation and stiffness. The Royal College of Midwives encourages a balanced exercise programme to improve posture and body awareness – this is essential as your centre of gravity shifts with the inevitable upward and outward change in your body. Exercising your pelvic floor muscles and abdominal wall muscles regularly will help them to regain strength and tone more quickly after delivery.

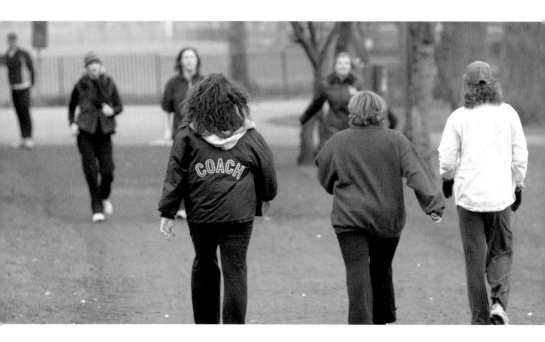

30s

After the age of 30 the body secretes less growth hormone, stimulating a loss of lean body tissue and encouraging greater storage of fat. In this decade, women lose 140–170g (5–6oz) of muscle mass a year and can gain as much, if not more, fat mass. If you are not doing any weight-bearing activity by the age of 39 you could potentially have lost 1.8kg (4lb) of muscle mass and replaced it with body fat, slowing your metabolism down still more, and putting you on the slippery road to further weight gain. Men are also likely to lose a lot of muscle mass in this decade if they don't maintain a high level of physical activity, and they are more prone to putting on weight round their abdomens (becoming apple-shaped).

40s

Peri-menopause is defined as the time leading up to menopause (it may start as early as ten years before menstruation ceases) and is marked by a fluctuation of hormones. Women at this stage experience a decrease in their metabolic rate owing to changes in hormones and muscle mass. Oestrogen levels become erratic, waxing and waning, and the storage site for fat shifts to your middle, around your abdomen. During peri-menopause many women experience mood swings, memory loss, bone loss, cholesterol changes, hot flushes and sleep disturbances, all of which may affect your self-esteem and motivation to keep physically active. Men will also notice signs of their metabolism decreasing.

50s

Menopause is defined as the 12 months after a woman's last period, usually around the age of 52. After menopause, women lose about 66 per cent of oestrogen and 50–60 per cent of testosterone. The oestrogen tends to decline at a faster rate than the testosterone and encourages a redistribution of body fat. In most cases, it is redistributed from the hips to the middle section and blood pressure and cholesterol levels rise. All these changes can put women at a higher risk of cardiovascular disorders, but it is overweight men who now find themselves in a real danger zone at this age. Consult your doctor before starting a new fitness or weight-loss programme in this age group.

60s+

Activity that focuses on balance, mobility and flexibility is especially important to help maintain posture and stability and safeguard against falls. Decline in physical activity levels with age is not inevitable and maintaining them can play an important part in the prevention of strokes, osteoporosis and arthritis. At this age, your daily nutritional energy needs start to lower as your muscle mass will be less than at younger ages.

However, getting a variety of food and maintaining your nutrient base is still vitally important, both for energy and for maintaining healthy weight. Daily walking and balance exercises can be simple but effective health investments for you and the quality of your life.

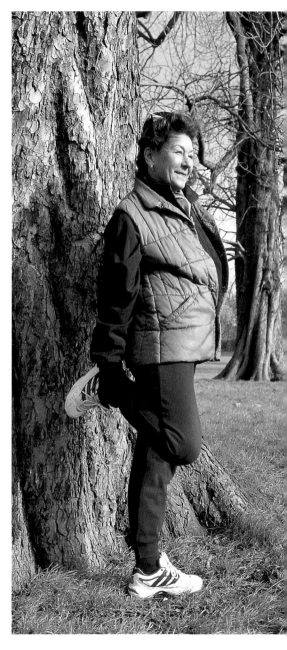

Action plans

Following is a quick reference guide for putting together an action plan to age-proof our bodies through the decades. You shouldn't wait till after 40 to begin looking after your body, but if you have, that's okay – remember that every little thing you do will make a difference. No matter how old or young you are, your body can still benefit from exercise.

IN YOUR 20s:

STOP... depriving yourself of water and sleep.

The niggling health problems that can make a misery of your 20s – such as headaches, eczema, depression, irritable bowel syndrome, bad skin and pre-menstrual syndrome (PMS) – often improve dramatically when you cut down on alcohol and junk food and increase your intake of water and sleep.

Water is a medium for the removal of all our waste products and the toxins that we put into our body. Aim to drink at least 2 litres/3½ pints a day. Sleep generates greater creativity and emotional balance, and improves short-term memory and problem-solving capabilities. Studies have also found that social drinkers who cut down on alcohol find themselves less anxious and depressed, and experience fewer mood swings.

START... getting into the exercise habit.

It may be a little while since you were playing sport at school, but don't let the absence of physical exercise become the norm. Get into the habit of taking regular structured exercise 2–3 times a week. Focus on cardiovascular activity to build up the stamina of your heart and lungs and to maintain your aerobic capacity. Experiment with mind-body exercise such as yoga to provide a balance in a perhaps frantic social life and boost body awareness.

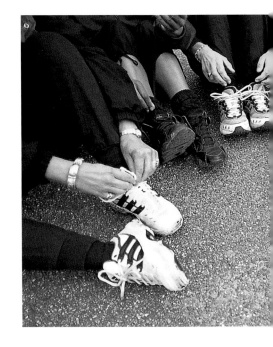

THINK ABOUT... the price of convenience.

Smoking (passive or active), convenience food and alcohol mean 20-somethings often end up with an antioxidant deficit. Antioxidants have been linked to the prevention of numerous conditions from heart disease and cancer to cataracts and arthritis. To rebalance, eat more fruit, vegetables and grains. Consider taking an antioxidant supplement (vitamins A, C and E, and minerals selenium, copper and zinc). Evening primrose oil can reduce pre-menstrual water retention and breast tenderness and vitamin B complex and magnesium may help with pre-menstrual problems that are more emotional than physical.

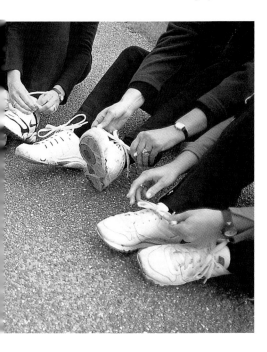

REMEMBER...

Women should go for regular cervical smears, and also a chlamydia test. Studies suggest that 1 in 20 sexually active women may have chlamydia.

IN YOUR 30s:

STOP... smoking.

If asthma, chest infections, bronchitis and various respiratory diseases haven't made you pack it in already, stop now! The risk of lung cancer increases exponentially if you have smoked for more than 20 years. As soon as you stop, your lungs start to recover.

START... to introduce some resistance exercise to your regular aerobic programme.

There are hundreds of reasons to exercise. Here are 5 to motivate you in your 30s.

1. Muscle mass starts to decline in your 20s, so you could be heading for an increase in your fat mass. If you are not doing weight bearing exercise, by age 39 you could potentially have lost 1.8kg/4lb of muscle mass and replaced it with body fat.

2. Fitter people have better circulation, which means a higher sex drive – important for women, who reach their sexual peak in their 30s.

3. Exercise is one of the most effective ways to control stress – whether you are a wife, mother or career-woman, the stresses of everyday life can be at their height right now.

4. The heart muscle needs exercise to remain strong. Staying fit lowers the risk of heart disease, diabetes and strokes, and raises oxygen levels in the body, keeping the brain alert.

5. Developing core strength through mind-body exercise such as Pilates will reduce your risk of back pain and help to maintain a lean, flat torso.

THINK ABOUT... stress levels.

Everyone needs space and solitude to relax. There are very few health problems – physical or mental – which are not related to stress. Find your stress outlet, whether it's yoga, swimming, walking or pottering about in the garden.

Vitamin B complex helps the functioning of the brain and nervous system. St John's wort can alleviate mild to moderate bouts of depression.

REMEMBER...

Check moles for changes in colour and shape.

IN YOUR 40s:

STOP... middle-age spread.

Insomnia, impotence, osteoporosis and diabetes are all linked to weight gain and inactivity. Lack of flexibility is one of the strongest indicators of ageing – so start a stretching programme and aim for at least 30 minutes' daily physical activity. This needs to become the foundation of your future health as moderate exercise has been shown to have the greatest impact on reducing blood pressure, insensitivity to glucose – an early indication of late-onset diabetes – and also on positively changing our blood lipid profile.

START... eating more fruit and fibre.

30–50 per cent of cancers are thought to be preventable if people adhered to a healthier diet. Bowel cancer, for example, is directly related to intake of fibre, fat and water. Heart disease is also strongly linked to diet: oily fish (fresh mackerel, tuna, salmon and tinned sardines) protect against heart disease by increasing beneficial high-density lipoproteins.

THINK ABOUT... fish oil and vitamin E supplements.

Fish oils help lower our blood cholesterol levels, improve circulation and ease arthritis. Vitamin E has also been linked with a reduced risk of prostate cancer and heart disease.

REMEMBER...

Ask your doctor to check your blood pressure and perhaps arrange a bone-density scan.

IN YOUR 50s:

STOP... standing on your bathroom scales!

Instead, monitor your body composition and specifically your body fat. You can use body fat monitoring devices in your home or at the gym. Muscle weighs more than fat, and while your weight may be similar to your weight in your 30s, your percentage body fat may have increased, placing you at greater risk of heart disease, diabetes and some cancers.

START... drinking 8 glasses of water a day.

By 50, our thirst mechanism can be suppressed, creating a situation where our body is chronically dehydrated, and even drinking 6 glasses of water a day instead of 8 can leave us chronically dehydrated. This has been linked to gall stones, kidney stones and bowel and prostate cancer.

THINK ABOUT... taking up t'ai chi.
Studies have shown that this discipline is one of the best ways to stimulate brain-eye co-ordination and improve body awareness. Studies on stroke victims found a significant improvement in recovery rates with regular t'ai chi.

REMEMBER... to have a regular health test.
Everyone should ask their doctor for a bowel cancer test, and women should have a mammogram every 3 years for the rest of their life. Those with a family history of breast or ovarian cancer may also want to be screened for ovarian cancer.

IN YOUR 60s:
STOP... doing high-impact workouts, and change your routine with more moderate and longer-duration exercise.
The risk of arthritis is greater, and more moderate, low-impact activity such as walking, swimming and t'ai chi will not place undue stress on the legs.

START... Mental exercises.
Never done the crossword at the back of the newspaper? Now is the time to start.

THINK ABOUT... having an annual flu jab, because flu can be far more dangerous when you are in your 60s.

REMEMBER...
To play with your grandchildren – and if you don't have grandchildren of your own, make a concerted effort to be amongst younger people. It will keep you both physically and mentally on the ball!

IN YOUR 70s:
START... to use your chronobiological rhythm!
Everyone has chronobiological highs and lows, and these relate to the physiological, psychological and cognitive functioning of our body. Take physical exercise when your body is on a down time and it will be harder to keep going and sustain motivation.

STOP... thinking this is it!
In a study of the 'super young', 3,500 people who seemed exceptionally young for their age found that one of the biggest contributing factors in retaining youthfulness was the continual development of friendships and interests.

THINK ABOUT... regularly measuring your blood pressure, either through your GP or with a home device.
High blood pressure can alert you to the danger of heart disease or strokes.

REMEMBER...
To have a bone scan to measure the density of your bones. In your 70s, you run a higher risk of fractures from falls.

Factors that may affect weight loss

It's possible that in the past you've found it unusually hard to shift those pounds. There may be reasons for this, and we'll have a look at some of them here. Understanding these forces can relieve the burden of guilt and point the way forward to effective weight-management solutions, strengthening the relationship between our brains and our bodies and weakening that Template of Failure.

GENES

We've already seen that our genes may account for up to 70 per cent of our body shape, which leaves about 30 per cent we can potentially change. This is because certain genes affect metabolism and/or eating behaviour, and therefore influence body mass and fat. They create a complex interplay of physiological processes that can affect our shape, rate of weight loss and appetite. While obesity is not inevitable, some people may be battling against a biological inheritance.

MODERN LIVING

It is now generally agreed that the fundamental causes of the obesity epidemic in the Western world are sedentary lifestyles and high-fat, energy-dense diets – products of the profound changes taking place in our society. The ever-increasing demands of the workplace mean that fewer people have time to cook fresh food; others are unaware of the hidden calories in convenience foods.

HUNGER DRIVE

Our appetite mechanism originated with our human forebears who lived in a harsh environment, hunting animals and gathering plants for food. They needed a healthy appetite – especially for calorifically dense foods – to ensure that they stored enough energy to keep them going through leaner times. This hunger drive was so essential for survival that some anthropologists believe there is an evolutionary residue, which, in the sedentary, food-rich Western world, often leads us to gain excess weight. It may not only affect our appetite but also regulate how efficiently we convert food into energy.

CALCIUM DEFICIENCY

One evolutionary factor associated with obesity is calcium levels. Studies by the US government, among others, show that people with higher levels of calcium have more control over their body weight. When calcium is abundant in the body, it appears that fat is used for energy. When calcium levels drop the body may shift into survival mode, encouraging increased fat storage.

INSULIN RESISTANCE

Hormones are complex molecules produced by the endocrine glands that manage many bodily functions and processes. Insulin, known as the 'hunger hormone', influences the amount of body fat we store by inhibiting food intake, increasing energy expenditure and regulating the amount of glucose (a sugar) in the blood. However, if a person is significantly overweight and consumes large amounts of refined ('simple') carbohydrates, this can result in the condition known as insulin resistance. A person with insulin resistance has to produce more insulin to reduce their blood glucose to normal levels, and so their satiety lever is never pushed (meaning they never feel full). Insulin resistance often leads to obesity, and both are major triggers of Type 2 diabetes.

STRESS HORMONES

Stress – whether physical or psychological – can wreak havoc with weight control by releasing the 'stress hormones' to deal with what the body perceives as an emergency. If stress is keeping you awake at night, your cortisol levels increase, encouraging the body to switch to a fat-storing mode. Studies have demonstrated that sleep deprivation increases both appetite and food consumption. If you don't think you can reduce your stress levels through exercise, or perhaps meditation, then see your doctor.

A TIME FOR YOU
One in four of us experiences depression at some point in our lives, and regular physical activity is one of the best depression busters around. I'm also a great believer that Structured Exercise is a time for you. We live in a fast-paced world, but Structured Exercise gives you little moments of 'me' time. It's an investment in yourself that no one can afford not to make.

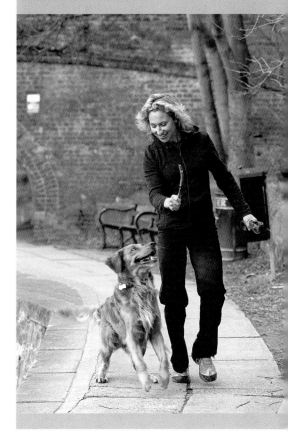

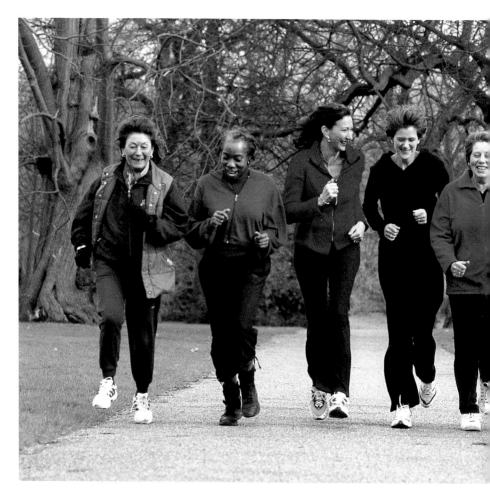

THE WINTER MONTHS

The time of year also may affect appetite. Many people
get depressed in the late autumn and winter, when
there is less sunlight, and often tend to eat more. This
condition is called Seasonal Affective Disorder (SAD).
Even those people who do not suffer from SAD are often
impelled by the colder weather to prefer heavy, hot foods
instead of salads.

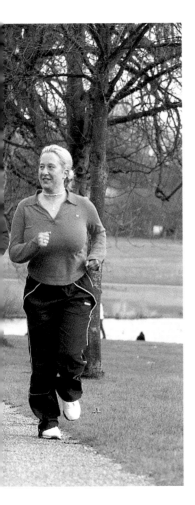

IS STRESS MAKING YOU FAT?

Some people thrive on stress, undertaking great challenges and reaching for the stars. Many of us, however, react to pressure by reaching for a bag of chocolate cookies. The relationship between stress and eating is complicated. Does stress simply reduce our willpower to make good food choices or does it actually increase our appetites?

The human stress response is intended as a short-term solution to an immediate problem, but we seldom face the kind of dangers that would require such a response. Our modern enemies are overloaded schedules, belligerent bosses, traffic jams, financial pressures and a host of other worries. They are formidable and can be deadly over the decades.

When faced with a stressful situation, our brains signal an acute immediate response causing the adrenal glands to release a hormone called cortisol. High levels of cortisol result in increased appetite and fat deposits. When stress is chronic and long-term, cortisol levels can remain elevated for long periods of time. This leads to increased body fat around the waist, higher blood pressure and blood sugar imbalances; further effects may include a vicious cycle of hormone imbalances linked to cardiac dysfunction and increased obesity.

Stress makes us crave foods that are calorie-laden and contain few nutrients. No definitive research has determined why stress-eaters make bad food choices. Some desire high-energy foods containing sugar, especially chocolate. Others prefer salty foods like crisps, chips, popcorn and crackers. Many overeat at the first signs of stress, while others initially shun food. However, after some initial weight loss from this reduction in food intake, approximately 40 per cent of people typically begin to eat excessively 6 to 7 weeks later, and ultimately weigh in above their original weight.

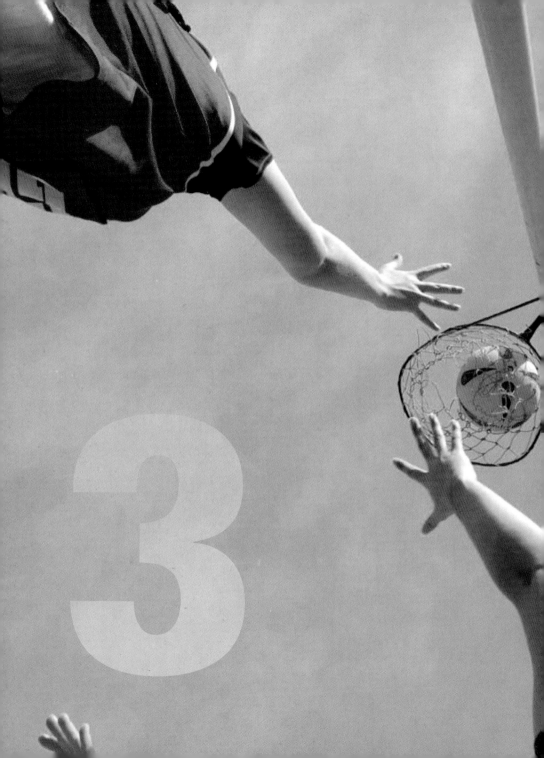

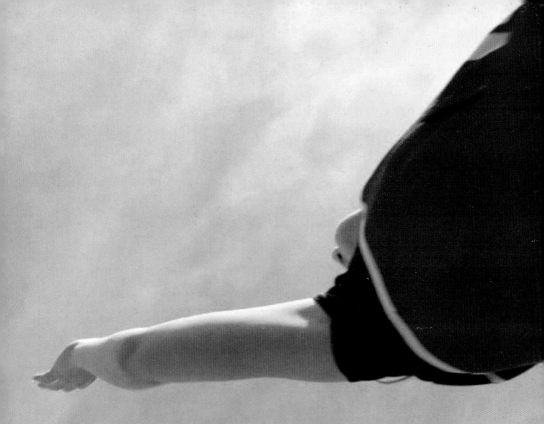

Making
it happen

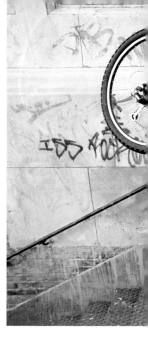

Maintaining
your weight loss

Most of what we know about people who have lost weight and kept it off comes from university-based weight-loss programmes, as few of the commercial programmes tend to collect or publish data.

The National Weight Control Registry is an American study founded in 1993 by professors at the University of Colorado and the University of Pittsburgh. Before they are signed up, dieters must have lost at least 14kg (30lb) each and have kept it off for minimum of a year. In fact, the average weight loss is 27kg (60lb) per person and they have kept it off for an average of 5 years – they like to be known as 'Successful Losers'. This makes them an extremely valuable group to study when formulating successful weight-loss strategies.

They all had four strategies in common:

- Eating a low-fat, high-carbohydrate diet of 1,300 to 1,500 calories per day (of which only 23 per cent to 24 per cent came from fat).
- Eating breakfast almost every day.
- Frequently monitoring their weight – this serves as an 'early warning system'.

- Maintaining a high level of physical activity. The mean energy they expended was 2,000 kcal a week for women and 3,300 kcal a week for men, with walking being the most popular form of exercise. This equates to about 60 to 90 minutes of moderate-intensity physical activity per day.

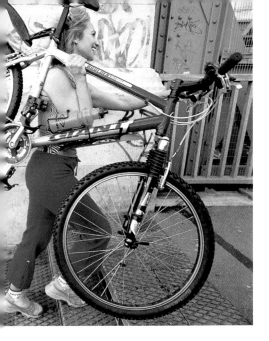

NAVIGATING YOUR DAY

The world of work can be frantic and stressful, and leave us very little time for ourselves – let alone an opportunity to take some structured exercise. Sometimes all we can do is hang on and hope we don't get tossed out along the way. The result? Energy-sapping, nerve-racking worry elevates our stress hormone (cortisol) levels. Research indicates that chronic exposure to elevated cortisol contributes to increased levels of fat deposition (specifically around our midriffs), which in turn is said to contribute to a 3–5-fold increase in the risk of certain diseases.

Day-in, day-out stress affects our posture and produces lethargy and body pain. From morning to evening our body's nervous system hits peaks and troughs as we cope with a barrage of demands:

deadlines, traffic jams, high-pressure meetings, the boss's moods and constant interruptions. Even when the ride is exhilarating, our nervous system still takes a battering. The human body was not designed for life on a roller-coaster. It is blasted with a constant bombardment of coffee, sugar, fast foods and snacks, and our inactive and sedentary lifestyle chained to a desk or with a telephone clamped to our ear compounds the problem. Instead of establishing a pleasant plateau of focus and energy in our life, we can find ourselves between frantic activity and sluggishness, as we experience adrenaline rushes, caffeine highs and blood glucose insulin rebounds.

But it does not have to be like this. If you are looking to even out the ride a bit, moving your body and making small changes to what you are eating and drinking can be hugely beneficial. Physical activity has been shown to be the best way to dissipate stress hormones. So here are some tips to help you become more stress-resilient and better prepared to cope with your daily work demands.

Even if your day doesn't revolve around an office and instead you have to cope with being at home with the kids, juggle a part-time job with your family commitments, or just lead a demanding social life, you can use the navigation path alongside as a guide to getting just a bit more activity into your day. Although not all the tips may be relevant, you can easily tailor them to fit your circumstances. Once they have become habits you will be more willing to experiment with others:

06.00: Arghh – the alarm goes off. This may not be your normal waking hour, but whatever time you get up, experiment with rising a little earlier and don't turn off your alarm. If you can't bring yourself to spring out of bed at the first alarm, place the clock so you have to S-t-r-e-t-c-h to turn it off. Don't stop there. Keep stretching, stretch through your fingers and all the way down to your toes while still lying in your bed. Look at any animal and you will see it always stretches itself as it wakes up. Movement stimulates the waking part of the brain so you will find it easier to escape the gravitational pull of the pillow!

06.15: Boil some water and make yourself a Wake-up Lemon Drink. Before you get dressed, try to fit in 3 or 4 Seated Sun Salutations as this will gradually raise your body temperature, which will have fallen during the night, and help your body's metabolism and enzyme activity. Sit, knees together, at the edge of a chair. Place your hands, palm together, at chest height. Inhale deeply and lift your arms out and up from your sides until they are directly above your head, palms touching, stretching up towards the sun. Exhale and relax your arms down to your sides.

WAKE-UP LEMON DRINK

Here's a drink that will wake up your excretory system. Boil a cup of water and mix it with the juice of a freshly squeezed lemon. Add a pinch of salt and, when the mixture is cool enough to drink, stir in up to a teaspoon of honey. The lemon juice cleanses the kidneys as well as the bowels, the salt will draw waste material from the bloodstream, and the honey soothes and tones the intestinal tract.

07.00: Skip the caffeine and substitute a glass of freshly squeezed, diluted orange juice or grapefruit juice. Bypass the sugary cereals, which create a fast sugar rush and then bring you crashing down, and opt instead for a slow-releasing breakfast option such as porridge oats with berries, a breakfast smoothie or a slice of toast with a boiled egg. No time to eat now? Then grab a flask and do a breakfast on-the-go smoothie.

08.00: Turn your commuting time into quiet time. If you drive, leave the radio off. If you commute, scan the papers selectively, check out the news-in-brief sections and then take a few moments to become aware of your breath and practise your 2:1 Breathing. You'll find you come into the office more refreshed and less frazzled, having had a little time to be still.

09.00: Resolve to walk briskly for at least 10 minutes before you sit down at your desk. As the pace picks up in the office, you will be pleased you have kick-started your body. In the next hour drink a glass of water, and eat your breakfast if you have brought it with you.

2:1 BREATHING

This breathing pattern relaxes the body by subtly coaxing the parasympathetic nervous system (which controls the automatic functions such as the beating of the heart and the digestion) into a state of relaxation.

Gently slow down the rate of exhalation until you are exhaling twice as long as you are inhaling. You can achieve longer exhalations by contracting the abdomen slightly. Don't try to fill or empty the lungs completely – it may help to count to 6 on the exhalation and 3 on the inhalation, or 4 on the exhalation and 2 on the inhalation (or any 2:1 ratio you find comfortable). Focus on the smoothness and evenness of your breath, gradually eliminating all jerks and pauses.

10.00: Quick posture check. Focus on how your body is positioned – it really won't take long. Check your feet are flat on the floor and you are extending through your spine, and consciously pull in your abdominal muscles to help keep the extension right up through your spine. Try to get up and move your body every 60 minutes – it will help stimulate blood flow to the brain and dissipate cortisol levels.

11.00: As your colleagues reach for that mid-morning caffeine and sugar fix, try to opt for a piece of fruit instead, although you may not be wanting it if you have had a nutritious breakfast. Drink some fruit juice as well as water, or try real ginseng tea or coffee substitutes, such as chicory.

12.00:
Do some neck stretches and rotate your spine; making sure you are sitting straight with your knees over your ankles, rotate your back so that you aim to look behind you. This will relieve tension in your upper body and reduce the compression through your lumbar vertebrae. If you have been working at a computer, try the Eyestrain Buster to energise your eye–brain communication.

EYESTRAIN BUSTER

This takes about 2 minutes and is great for relieving strained, tired eyes. Open your hands and gently slide the undersides of the thumbs across the upper rim of the eye sockets towards the temples. Then massage the lower rim of the eye sockets with your index fingers. Begin at the corners of your eyes and work towards the temples. Repeat twice more.

Now move your eyes slowly from side to side 3 times, slowly up and down 3 times, and finally in complete circles. Relax by closing your eyes so gently the eyelids barely touch.

13.00:
Try to avoid working through your lunch break. Even if you have a deadline to hit, don't skip your lunch. You need to eat something to replenish vital blood glucose – essential to help you concentrate – and a quick walk will help reduce your cortisol levels. So when you go out, make sure you walk for at least 10 minutes before you buy your lunch. Lunch can sap your energy, so select a meal that combines several proteins, as this will stimulate the brain transmitter dopamine that makes us feel more alert, as well as some starch, which fuels our muscles' glycogen levels. Avoid too heavy a food intake, as this will drain your energy levels and leave you craving a sugar and caffeine fix to kick-start your afternoon.

14.00:
You're back at your desk. Make sure that you drink a glass of water in the next hour. Reassess your posture and ensure that your shoulder blades are down and there is a good distance between your ears and your shoulders. Check your breathing, and make sure you are allowing the air to enter all the way into the body down to the diaphragm as chest breathing automatically triggers the nervous system.

15.00:
Starting to slump? Complete whatever you are in the middle of, then get up and move your body – even if that only means climbing a set of stairs or walking to the post box. You will return to your desk feeling more positive and able to continue with your 'To Do' list with renewed vigour. Can't get away from your desk?

INTRODUCE THE 5PM CARB CURFEW

Carb Curfew means no starchy carbs – bread, pasta, rice, potatoes or cereal – after 5pm. Don't panic – you won't feel as if you're about to starve, since you can incorporate a whole variety of nutritious foods in your evening meal, including lean meat and fish, fruit, vegetables, pulses and dairy products, and come up with something absolutely delicious!

Many of my clients consider the Carb Curfew to be the single most important tool in their weight management success and I know it can help you too. The Carb Curfew helps you control your insulin levels, which means it's easier to stabilise your energy levels – important for weight loss.

Why?

■ It's an easy way to create an Energy Gap! You will be cutting down on calories and filling up slow-releasing, energy-providing pulses, so you'll feel less hungry and more energetic.
■ Substituting fruit and vegetables instead of rice or pasta will increase your vitamin and mineral intake, which is important for the breakdown of macronutrients.
■ It reduces bloating. As your body digests and stores carbohydrate, it breaks it down into glucose and either stores it as glycogen in the muscles or as fat in the fat cells. Storing those starchy carbs as glycogen is your body's preferred choice but to do this it has to store three units of water with every one unit of glycogen. The net result is a bloated tummy.
■ If you stuff your face at night, you wake up with a 'food hangover' and won't want breakfast. By the evening, you'll be starving again.

Then lower your chest to your thighs, link your arms under them, hold on at the elbows or forearms and pull up through the upper back. This relieves tension in the upper back and shoulder area.

16.00. The classic vending-machine hour! Resist the urge for that sugar fix, but do allow yourself to eat a strategic snack if you feel hungry. Opt for something that will hydrate you, and that contains a little protein and natural sugar. Try a ginseng tea and a bio yoghurt, or a fruit smoothie, that will help curb your body's hunger pangs later.

17–18.30. Your journey home can be a challenging battle with those hunger pangs. As you walk out of the office, focus on your posture: make sure you extend up through your spine. If you really can't resist the quick-fix snack urge, walk briskly for 10 minutes before you buy anything. And make sure it is always a bottle of water first!

19.00. This is your time to get a little hot and sweaty in your structured exercise. If you tend to overeat at night, and especially if you have had a stressful day, focus on increasing the intensity of your workout efforts, even if this means reducing the length of your

STOPPING PORTION DISTORTION – A FEW TIPS

Weighing out the correct portion of food can be a bore, so let's make things simple. To keep your meals in check, compile a handy Portion Distortion basket in your kitchen. Put in it some everyday items that are the same size as the portion of food you should be eating. Soon you'll become familiar with the sizes, so in a restaurant you can order what you want but only eat as much as the size of the healthy portion. You can still eat the foods you like, so you don't feel deprived, but you have control over what you consume and the number of calories you take in. Use the following objects to judge the portion size you should be aiming at.

Think...	For...
Two dice	Nuts and cheese
Deck of cards	Meat and fish
Teaspoon	Oils and fats
Tennis ball	Vegetables
Golf ball	Uncooked rice or coucous
Computer mouse	Cooked portion of starchy carbs

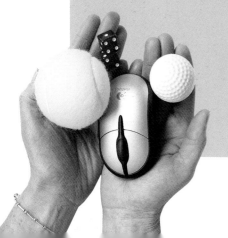

exercise session. Thirty minutes is all you need. Studies have shown that exercising at a higher intensity will actually suppress your appetite and decrease your levels of cortisol. In addition, current evidence suggests that exercising at varying intensities is far more beneficial in terms of weight loss than always working at a slow pace for a longer time.

20.00: Your evening meal should include fresh vegetables, fruit, some grains and good-quality protein such as fish, lean meat and pulses. Try to have a range of colours on your plate: this will provide a rich variety of nutrients and boost your antioxidant intake. Whatever you choose, try to keep it light, especially if you eat late. A heavy meal before bed will interfere with your sleep and you will feel sluggish when you need to wake up.

21–22.00: Try to unwind with a relaxing activity. If you have a family, play a game or team up to prepare tomorrow's lunch or breakfast.

23.00: How you go to sleep has everything to do with how you wake up. If you experience difficulty sleeping, try the Meditation or Systematic Relaxation before getting into bed. Once in bed, try the Sleep Exercise.

MEDITATION

The practice of meditation gently frees us from the worries and mental entanglements that gnaw away at our body as we respond to the needs of the moment. It does not have to be time-consuming. Even a few moments in the morning and 5 minutes in the evening before bed will calm the nervous system and soothe the mind. Find a quiet, private place. Sit on the floor with a cushion under you or in a firm chair, with your head and back straight and your eyes closed. Allow all your muscles to relax except those that are supporting your head, neck and back.

When your body is relaxed, bring your awareness to your breath. Let it come primarily from the diaphragm, leaving your chest and shoulders motionless. Experience your breathing in an open and accepting way. As thoughts come let them pass without reacting to them and continue to be aware of your breath. Gently repeat the words 'I am perfectly still' in your mind.

SYSTEMATIC RELAXATION

This is a great way to clear your mind of tension. It reduces stress while resting the mind and body. With constant practice you can learn to relax in the space of a few breaths. Lie on your back with a small pillow under your head, your palms up and your feet slightly spread. Allow the floor to support you and turn your attention to your breath for a few moments. Then mentally scan the body from head to toe and back again, pausing briefly to become aware of each area. Aim to release any tension you notice. Begin with the top of the head, then move to the forehead, face, jaws and ears. Continue to the throat, shoulders, upper arms, palms, fingers and fingertips. Return along the joints of the wrist, elbows and shoulders. Relax the spine, abdomen and pelvis, the buttocks, thighs, calves, shins, feet, toes and toe tips. Exhale and inhale 4 times as though your whole body is exhaling and inhaling. Exhale all your worries and anxieties. Inhale vital energy, tranquillity and peace.

Become aware of the joints of the toes, the ankles, knees and hips. Relax the vertebrae from the coccyx to the base of the neck. Relax the head and the top of the head. Exhale from the head to the tips of the toes and inhale from the toe tips back to the top of the head. Repeat this 3 times. Be aware of the calm flow of the breath. Make a gentle effort to guide your breath so that it remains smooth and deep without jerks or pauses. Gently open your eyes. Stretch and notice how you feel. Try to maintain this feeling of calmness.

SLEEP EXERCISE

This great little technique will not only get you off to sleep but also help you sleep more peacefully. It uses an effortless 2:1 breath. Pay close attention to your breathing. There should not be any pauses, jerks or shakiness. Eliminate even the pause between the inhalation and exhalation.

Get into bed and take:
8 breaths lying on your back;
16 breaths lying on your right side;
32 breaths lying on your left side.
Very few people complete this exercise. Sweet dreams!

Barrier Bashing

I'm sure you remember that barrier bashing involves identifying what you think may pose a challenge to your efforts, and then a little problem-solving and planning ahead to devise ways of bashing it down, so that you can continue on your journey. Once you've developed strategies to keep up your sleeve, you can always prevent or at least minimise a potential challenge.

Below is a list of some of the barriers I have come across with my clients, along with solutions we devised, and I hope that you will find them useful too. Of course, you'll have some barriers that are unique to you, and you'll have to invent strategies for bashing them down yourself.

BARRIER: ARRIVE HOME STARVING!

This is one of the most common times when people get into trouble with those addictive foods.

Bash it down: Have a snack after work, because this will take the edge off your hunger and may help stop you over-eating at dinner too. Make sure you have a ready supply of fruits, nuts, or other non-trigger foods in the house that you put aside especially for this time. Alternatively, stop off at a coffee shop on the way home and instead of ordering a large coffee, have a large cup of skimmed milk to curb your hunger.

PARTY TIME!

Parties can present a tricky barrier on your weight-loss journey – but they don't have to be your downfall. With a little navigation and pre-planning, you can go to the ball!

ALTERNATIVE SNACKS

Instead of...	Choose...
2 sausage rolls (480 calories)	3 cocktail sausages (260 calories)
30g slice of quiche (141 calories)	a 90g chicken drumstick (130 calories)
28g of salami (120 calories)	28g turkey breast (35 calories)
4 glasses of red wine (380 calories)	4 white wine spritzers (200 calories)
Scooping your dips with crackers, breadsticks, pitta bread and tortilla chips (365 calories)	Scoop your dips with crudités (1 calorie per vegetable stick)
a packet of crisps (150 calories)	a pack of Twiglets (95 calories)
4 After Eights (140 calories)	4 satsumas (100 calories)
6 chocolate brazil nuts (330 calories)	6 dates (90 calories)

THE LOWDOWN ON LIQUID CALORIES

Liquid calories can easily add up, but with some wise choices you can still enjoy a drink or two without it throwing your whole weight-loss strategy off balance. Space out your alcoholic drinks by having a large glass of water in between.

Drink	Liquid calories
1 x 275ml bottle low-alcohol lager	40
1 medium sherry	60
1 port	70
1 x 175ml glass of orange juice	70
1 x 275ml bottle Pils	75
1 gin and diet tonic	85
1 x 125ml glass dry white/red wine	85
1 x 125ml glass of champagne	95
1 half pint lager	100
1 Pimms and lemonade	110
1 x 125ml glass sweet white wine	118
1 rum and coke	123
1 x 330 ml glass Pina Colada	486

Four great party tricks

- Eat before you go out. Plan your snacks so you don't arrive at the party starving – it will be your biggest downfall. Remember to keep well hydrated right through the day of your party, too, as this can help minimise hunger and the effects of a heavy night.
- Know your dips. Go for salsa ones (5 calories per 10g scoop) or tsatziki (10 calories per 10g scoop). They're lower in calories (and fat) than creamy dips, such as sour cream or taramasalata.
- Try 'spicy' drinks. A tomato juice with a dash of Tabasco sauce won't stimulate your appetite nearly as much as sweeter drinks (whether they're alcoholic or not).
- Don't stand anywhere near the bowls of crisps and nuts or you'll end up grazing all evening.

Festive fare at home

- Eat your mince pies topless! If you have a mince pie fetish at Christmas time, go for the ones without the pastry lid: they only have 160 calories, while ordinary mince pies weigh in at over 200 calories. And, if you usually eat them with cream (170 calories per 45g), try low-fat fromage frais (35 calories per 30g) instead.
- Eat your Christmas cake naked! An average slice will set you back about 418 calories. Take off the icing and marzipan, however, and you'll save yourself about 239 calories.

BARRIER: STRESS MAKES ME CRAVE CARBS!

Carbs trigger the production of a feel-good hormone called serotonin, which helps to boost your mood and temporarily relieve your stress.

Bash it down: Give in to a carb-rich lunch occasionally. Using food for temporary relief from a problem is fine as long as you don't do it all the time. Plan your menus in a way that allows you to enjoy chicken nuggets with potato wedges every now and then. Better still, try to eat a very small portion of carbs along with a high-protein food such as steak, chicken or tuna salad. Stride out stress as well – when really stressed, go out for a brisk, 15-minute, stress-busting walk.

BARRIER: THE 4 O'CLOCK CHOCOLATE HOUR

Your energy levels are low and you are slumping big-time – chocolate seems the only answer!

Bash it down: Give in – but just a little. If you have an intense craving for a very specific food – like chocolate (and remember, chocolate contains an addictive, mood-altering substance) – I think it's best to go ahead and eat it. If you don't, your craving is going to get more intense until you eventually give in anyway and you will have consumed a lot of unnecessary calories in your attempt to make it go away. Have a glass of milk and 2 cubes of dark chocolate, and make sure

you don't wolf it down as this is all about making you feel more in control.

If you do succumb to biscuits, make sure you keep the lapse under control – meaning take two or three biscuits or pieces of chocolate at most, and then put the rest away. You may feel as if you want more but it's worth knowing that, according to a study conducted at Pennsylvania State University, people who were served the smallest portions of a food felt just as full and satisfied as those who were given unlimited helpings of the same food.

If you do lapse big-time, then make a note of it when you review your week and think of an appropriate contingency plan you could use to redress the balance.

BARRIER: EVENING CRISP CRAVING

In the evening you want to relax. The crisp craving that strikes at this time is less about the food and more about what the food signifies – chilling out and maybe rewarding yourself after a tough day.

Bash it down: Fight the urge to eat – you are eating for the wrong reason. When it happens too often, this kind of emotionally driven eating becomes a primary reason for weight gain. To break the habit, bite the bullet and go cold turkey – no food while the TV's on. Create food-free zones, such as 6.30–8pm, since even healthy snacks won't help break the association between food and relaxing. To make the process easier, decide to do something during that time that doesn't involve sitting down, such as rearranging the living-room furniture. Studies suggest that hanging out in the same spot where you have indulged past cravings can trigger new ones.

BARRIER: PRE-BED ICE-CREAM URGE

This is a fairly natural urge, since carbohydrates help to boost levels of a sleep-inducing compound called tryptophan. As tryptophan levels in your brain increase, you become sleepier.

Bash it down: Say no! Opt for a glass of warm milk or a low-calorie hot chocolate drink. Alternatively, say yes! No, you're not misreading this; if saying no just doesn't work, go ahead and give in to the ice-cream. Better that than hunger keeping you awake. Keep the serving small and pick a regular, full-fat ice-cream – not the fat-free kind, because you may well end up eating more of it. According to a study from Purdue, taste buds can detect fat and that may be why fat-free foods aren't as satisfying as full-fat foods.

BARRIER: I'M STILL HUNGRY AFTER DINNER!

This may be because you are eating too quickly rather than not eating enough. It takes 20 minutes for the stretch receptors in your stomach lining to send a message to the brain registering food – by that time, you may have eaten well beyond your calorie needs. Eating too quickly can cause digestive problems and is thought to be a cause of irritable bowel syndrome.

Bash it down: Time how long it takes you to eat each meal. Then try to give yourself longer to finish each one, starting off by aiming to increase your recorded time by 50 per cent for one whole week. The following week, try to add a further 50 per cent. Eat until you are 80 per cent full. You know what 100 per cent full feels like, so stop short before you get to that point. Persevere with this – it allows your brain to become aware of how food feels as it starts to enter your body, stopping you from over-eating and actually energising you more. Eating too much food decreases your immediate energy levels, as your body has to work harder to digest your food. Stopping short of finishing should also empower you, as you'll feel more in control of your food volume.

INSTEAD OF A 250-CALORIE CHOCOLATE BAR, SELECT ONE OF THE FOLLOWING 100 CALORIE SNACKS:

2 squares Dairy Milk chocolate

2 oatcakes

any piece of fruit

20 almonds

8 dried apricots

1 small pot low-fat yoghurt

a palmful of sunflower and pumpkin seeds

2 rice cakes topped with cottage cheese

half a small avocado filled with salsa

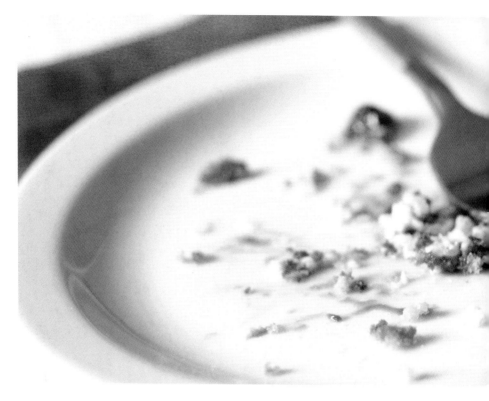

BARRIER: I'M GOING OUT TO DINNER

You must have realised by now that I firmly believe living a healthy, balanced life includes going out and having a good time. You don't have to put your weight-loss journey on hold just because some friends invite you for an evening out.

Bash it down: Instead of sticking to your Carb Curfew dinner and causing all sorts of complications for your host, have a starch curfew lunch instead. This allows you to include some starch with your evening meal without over-indulging.

This one's a useful strategy for those of us who over-eat when away from our home territory. Divide the food

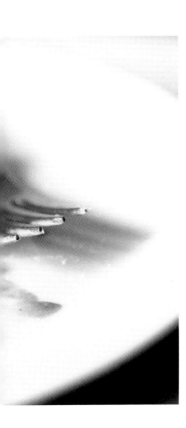

on your plate in two halves. If you are dining out, you can make an imaginary line. Eat half the food. Stop for 10 minutes and either leave the table, or sip a glass of water until it's empty.

If you are still hungry after 10 minutes, finish your meal. If you are not sure, divide the remainder in half and repeat the exercise in exactly the same way.

Order first, drink later. Alcohol loosens your inhibitions, making you less careful when ordering. It also leaves you feeling less satisfied after your meal, resulting in an increased calorie intake over the next 24 hours.

My usual, please! If you're going to a restaurant that you know, decide beforehand what you would like to order. That way, you won't be tempted by high-calorie specials when you open the menu. There are tips on dishes to opt for in different kinds of restaurant on pages 72–3.

How to survive eating out

If you're afraid to eat out in case your good intentions and resolve weaken when you're confronted with an exciting restaurant menu, don't be. All you have to do is try to stick to the low-fat, vitamin-rich menu choices outlined over the page. The golden rule is to avoid anything fried, as this will be overloaded with fat – and our fat cells love to feed on fatty foods. Remember, as well, to apply the Carb Curfew where possible – but if you really want some carbs, you can shift your Curfew to the middle of your day so that lunch becomes your Carb-Free Zone!

AT SOCIAL EVENTS:

Alcohol, soft drinks, cheesy snacks, bread, sweets and other common trigger foods are likely to be offered. Before you head out, eat a handful of nuts, a piece of fruit or another non-trigger food, or make yourself a smoothie before you go.

READ THAT MENU CAREFULLY

British menus

- Ask for a prawn cocktail without the dressing.
- Minestrone and consommé are low-fat starters.
- If you're allowing yourself carbs, choose boiled or jacket potatoes instead of roast.
- Skip the gravy – choose mint sauce, mustard or herb seasonings instead.
- Don't eat the skin on roast chicken or duck.
- Request plain vegetables without butter.
- Avoid cooked breakfasts; cereal is a lower-fat option.

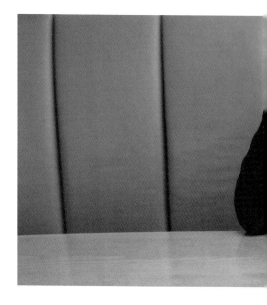

American menus

- Choose a restaurant with a self-service salad bar.
- Avoid pre-dressed salads and instead dress your own with seasoned vinegars, or lemon juice and herbs.
- Use mayonnaise, ketchup and relishes sparingly.
- Choose baked potatoes instead of chips and don't add butter or sour cream.

Indian menus

- Curries can be very high in fat; choose vegetable options and avoid dishes like chicken korma, which contain cream.
- Indian flat breads are a good choice and better than poppadoms, which are deep-fried.
- Basmati rice is an excellent option.
- Avoid deep-fried onion and vegetable bhajis.

Chinese menus

- Fried rice is very high in fat; choose boiled rice which has almost no fat at all.
- Request boiled noodles instead of fried noodles.
- Tofu (bean curd) is a low-fat protein option that is found in many oriental dishes.
- Stir-fried vegetables are a good choice.
- Don't be tempted to snack on prawn crackers – they are deep-fried so have a high fat content.
- Avoid spring rolls – these also contain a great deal of fat.
- Cashew nuts are high in saturated fat.
- Beansprouts and water chestnuts are a good option.
- Lychees are an excellent, low-fat choice for dessert.

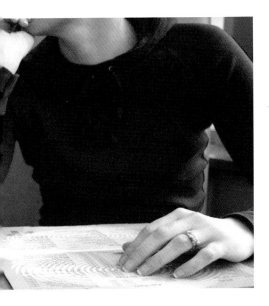

Italian menus

- Minestrone soup, melon and trimmed Parma ham are low-fat starters.
- Skinless breast of chicken and grilled fish dishes are a good choice.
- Choose a simple tomato sauce for pasta and only add a small sprinkling of Parmesan cheese.
- Avoid high-fat carbonara, cream or cheese sauces.
- Chargrilled vegetables or seafood are a tasty, low-fat option – but watch for the excessive use of olive oil, which can often be deceptive.
- Choose sorbet or fresh fruit instead of ice-cream for dessert.
- Cappuccino coffee can add extra unnecessary calories; opt for mint or camomile tea instead; alternatively, if caffeine is a necessity, an espresso is a better choice.

Japanese menus

- Miso soup with noodles and vegetables is a good choice.
- Sasami and seaweed salad is an excellent choice, rich in protein, essential fats and iodine.
- Soba noodles, made with buckwheat, are low in fat.
- Nori rolls (rice wrapped in seaweed) are deliciously low-calorie.
- Boiled rice is better than high-fat fried rice.
- Chicken or beef teriyaki and raw fish sushi or sashimi are also good, low-fat choices.

Middle Eastern menus

- Taboulleh salad made with cracked wheat and herbs is good choice.
- Houmous (made without cream) and yoghurt dips served with pitta breads are healthy options.
- Try to avoid taramasalata, as this can be a hidden calorie holder.
- Vine leaves stuffed with raisin rice, couscous dishes and savoury lentils are all good choices.
- Avoid deep-fried falafel, fatayer and samosas.
- Opt for baba ganoush (puréed aubergines with lemon juice), kebabs served with salad, shashlik (marinated meat or veg on a skewer) or grilled meat and fish dishes.

73

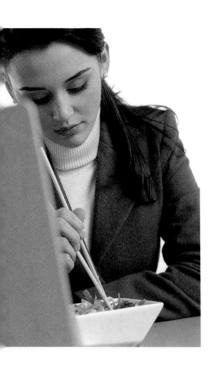

BARRIER: WE DON'T HAVE TIME FOR PROPER DINNERS

Not eating as a family can cultivate some bad eating habits for everyone – one survey showed that overweight children ate at least half of their meals in front of the television. Others revealed that youngsters who had dinner with their parents ate lower-fat foods, chose more fruit and vegetables, and were less prone to anxiety and depression, regardless of their social background.

Bash it down: Make a family dinner date. Mark everyone's calendars and tell them their attendance at dinner is requested. You could even write invitations to make it more of a special occasion.

If time's definitely your problem, bring home healthy fast food. Try pre-cut, frozen, canned or microwave-in-the-bag veg. Turn up the nutrition on canned soups by adding frozen vegetables and pre-cooked chicken breasts. Dig out the slow cooker. Toss in frozen chicken breasts, a bag of frozen carrots, chopped onions and a jar of low-salt sauce before you leave for work. Your meal will be ready when you get home.

Sit down on the run. If you only have time for a quick bite at a fast-food restaurant you can still make it a healthy affair. For example, choose grilled chicken with no sauce and remove the skin, or a single burger with lettuce and tomato instead of a triple cheeseburger. Order side salads (hold the dressing) and skip the fizzy drinks, opting instead for low-fat milk, water and juice. Unfortunately, pizza can be a minefield, laden with cheese, high-fat meat and oil. The main problem, however, is the size of the helping you're usually given. If you're eating out, share a pizza with a friend and fill up with a side salad. Or ask the restaurant to use half the usual amount of cheese, substituting it for a variety of vegetable toppings.

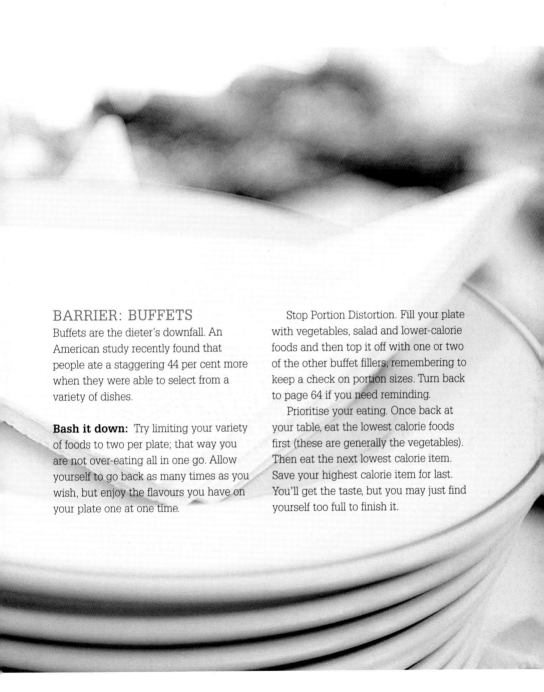

BARRIER: BUFFETS

Buffets are the dieter's downfall. An American study recently found that people ate a staggering 44 per cent more when they were able to select from a variety of dishes.

Bash it down: Try limiting your variety of foods to two per plate; that way you are not over-eating all in one go. Allow yourself to go back as many times as you wish, but enjoy the flavours you have on your plate one at one time.

Stop Portion Distortion. Fill your plate with vegetables, salad and lower-calorie foods and then top it off with one or two of the other buffet fillers, remembering to keep a check on portion sizes. Turn back to page 64 if you need reminding.

Prioritise your eating. Once back at your table, eat the lowest calorie foods first (these are generally the vegetables). Then eat the next lowest calorie item. Save your highest calorie item for last. You'll get the taste, but you may just find yourself too full to finish it.

BARRIER: WEEKENDS

When there's less of a routine, you let it all go.

Bash it down: Try the two-meal tool. At weekends, we often have two meals quite close together. Many of us have breakfast late and then lunch an hour or two later. Both these meals will also tend to be a bit bigger than you would have during the week. Save calories by having just two meals a day at weekends, breakfast (or brunch) and dinner, and just a snack in between.

Cook on a full stomach. If you have to bake or prepare for a dinner party, try to do it when you are full, after a meal or in the morning. You'll be less inclined to nibble.

Stretch your lunch. If you know you always get hungry in the afternoon, split your lunch into two sittings. Eat half at your normal lunchtime and the remaining half in the afternoon – but make sure you sit down for it rather than eating it at the fridge.

BARRIER: MENSTRUAL CYCLE

Many women find that, try as they might, they just can't resist those food cravings before and/or during a period. This is quite natural – studies show that in the two weeks leading up to your period, your metabolic rate actually increases by about 140 calories. The problem is that the chocolate bar you are craving will, on average, provide 250 calories.

Bash it down: If you really feel you are not going to be able to resist a binge, allocate a binge zone of up to a couple of hours. This is a time when you allow yourself to binge, but eat your fill of the lowest-calorie foods possible – try bowls of water-packed fruits or some steamed veg. You will fill yourself up, but stay within your calorie limit. If you still lapse, then take it on the chin and adopt a contingency plan the following day.

BARRIER: I FEEL POWERLESS TO STOP MYSELF

If you are binge-eating regularly, you need to work on your Template of Success, and you might like to start by revisiting the steps to self-esteem on pages 12–15. In the meantime, the following tips might help at the moment the urge strikes.

Bash it down: Take time out, and disconnect temporarily from everything food-related. Remember: you are in control, but you need to give yourself some space to realise this. Get up from the table, brush your teeth, or stop and clean a room in the house. Do whatever it takes to give yourself a break.

Switch the taste sensation. You can help stop a binge in its tracks by switching to a completely different food the moment you catch yourself at the point of bingeing. So, if you have started to polish off a carton of ice-cream, put the carton away and pull out a bag of fruit or carrot sticks. It will give you an opportunity to create some distance from the easy-eating, high-calorie food.

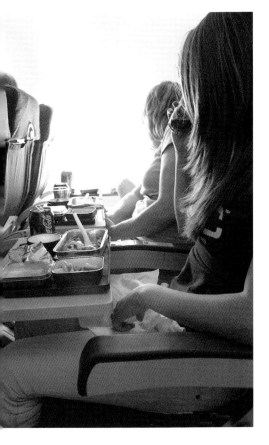

BARRIER: I TRAVEL SO MUCH

Being away from your normal environment can be a killer. Your routine is shot to pieces, you mainly eat out, you may have to decipher different food cultures, and, of course, you're just plain tired.

Bash it down: Pre-order your aeroplane meal. Most airlines are quite happy to do this, but they tend not to make it public knowledge. There is a wide range of special meals you can order – low fat, low calorie, low cholesterol, kosher, vegetarian, to name a few. Watch out for the veggie option, as it is almost invariably high in fat. I'd recommend you request a low-calorie rather than the low-fat meal as I have found the latter often turns out to be a low-cholesterol meal that still has a high fat content. And remember to say no to the bread roll and drink plenty of water.

Plan some prior protein! Make sure your last pre-travel meal contains a good balance of protein and starch, so you feel

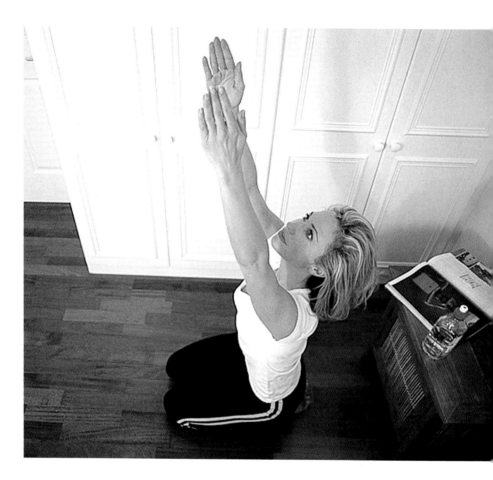

satisfied and motivated. Athletes journeying to international competitions use this strategy to minimise the detrimental effects of travelling on their performance. Before a long drive, have less protein but with lots of vegetables and fruit. Remember not to eat too much or your blood sugar levels will rise too quickly and you'll feel lethargic.

Blinker out the sweets at the garage counter. If you must buy something, grab some chewing gum and a bottle of water.

Pack your pedometer. You may not feel like exercising as soon as you arrive at your destination but do try to move your body – resolve to get 4,000 steps on that pedometer as soon as possible.

It's a great way to explore, and it'll help you get rid of travel fatigue. If you are on a business trip and your structured exercise sessions are just not going to happen, resolve to get in your daily 10,000 steps – even if it means getting up a little earlier.

Avoid excess baggage! If you are at a bar, or are offered nibbles with your pre-dinner drink, say NO – they are laden with salt and calories. Implement a Carb Curfew wherever possible.

It works at home and it works just as well when you're away. Try varieties of fruit and vegetables that aren't available at home, and restrict starchy foods to lunchtimes.

LIFESTYLE AND OCCUPATIONAL ACTIVITY

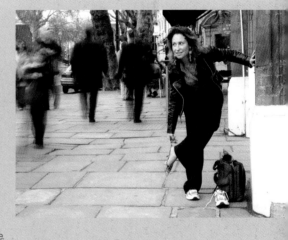

As we know, Structured Exercise – sport, or going to the gym, for example – has a major role to play in your overall energy expenditure but we also know that it's not the only way to burn off calories. Your body expends energy every time it moves, so your day-to-day activities, whether at work (Occupational Activity) or in your own time (Lifestyle Activity), all contribute to weight loss. Understanding this can inspire everyone to invent ways of incorporating more physical activity into their daily routine.

Remember: your fat cells will not be able to differentiate between a machine at the gym and a flight of stairs at work. The more you move your body, and the more energetically you move it, the greater amount of energy your body will burn and the more weight it will lose.

HOW CAN I DO IT?

Remember: all calories count, independent of the intensity of the activity. If you reduce the time you spend on sedentary things like watching TV, you will free up time for more active pursuits. Small changes such as this, systematically incorporated into your lifestyle, can have a big impact on the metabolism. In practical terms you can achieve your target by accumulating more steps throughout your day as well as taking more vigorous structured exercise.

Treat yourself

Glamorous Gym Locations

BERLIN
Oasis Fitness Gesundheitszentrum
When packing your suitcase don't forget your Badenhosen, as the highlight of this club is the Olympic-sized pool. If you really want to know what it feels like to swim 100m in Olympic time, here is your chance! If swimming is not your thing, break sweat in the well-equipped gym or with less effort in one of the 3 saunas. As it's open till 10pm, there really is no excuse for being a couch potato once you've finished that business report!
Stresemannstrabe, 74 Kreuzberg, Berlin, Germany
Tel: (+49) 262 6661

BRUSSELS
Champneys
The one thing you just must do at this club is to have the aqua massage. You don't even have to get wet: you just lie down fully clothed as you enjoy the sensation of water jets pummelling your body through super-dry plastic covering. And if that is not enough to leave you feeling refreshed, there's piped music in the relaxation rooms, and plunge pools and therapies to try out before you sweat away your day in the state-of-the-art gym. If you are a regular European traveller and a member of Champneys hospitality free of charge in London too.
Champneys Brussels, Avenue Louise 71B,
1050 Brussels, Belgium
Tel: (+32) 02 542 46 66

LONDON
The Third Space
Kitted out with the latest top-of-the-range fitness equipment, this £13 million health temple is the darling of the media fraternity in London's trendy Soho area. The runners and bikers have their own personal MP3 players and are netted up to surf, e-mail and watch mpegs as they pound the flesh. A 75m/245ft climbing wall may prove a challenge for some, or you can go several rounds with your own military trainer in the competition-sized boxing ring. If you don't fancy that, you can always get some serious run-training in the high-altitude run chamber. And the 20m/65ft pool is treated with ozone, not chlorine, so you won't get sore eyes!
13 Sherwood Street, London W1
Tel: (+44) 020 7439 6333

MILAN
Club 10 Health and Beauty
This laid-back club is more the place to be seen than the place to break sweat. Located in one of Milan's grandest hotels, the beautiful setting boasts a well-equipped gym for beautiful people. Supermodels mostly prefer to swim a few laps of the bijou swimming pool or pummel their stress away in the

whirlpool before indulging in the sauna, steam and beauty rooms for treatments.
Hotel Principe di Savoia, Milan, Italy
Tel: (+39) 02 62301

NEW YORK

Chelsea Piers Complex

Your family will need a week rather than day to enjoy the extensive all-lifestyle facilities at the Pier. The Sports Club at Pier 60 is renowned as the best gym in the world, and for good reason. Why not practise your running technique on the 3km/1.8 mile indoor running track while taking in the breathtaking views across the Hudson River? With two exercise studios (boasting over 150 classes a week, ranging from 'urban yoga' to 'warrior girl workouts'), a Pilates machine studio, boxing ring, volleyball courts, and a huge pool, you will be quite ready to lounge on the sundeck before going off to ice skate, rock climb, go-kart… Better still, head for a relaxation treatment at the Origins Spa located inside.
Pier 60 at 23rd Street at the West Side Highway, New York City, USA
Tel: (+1) 212 336 6262

SAO PAOLO

Centro de Practicas Esportivas de Universidade de Sao Paolo

If you go for a workout here, you may leave bemoaning the fact that facilities like these were unimaginable when you were at school! This phenomenal university illustrates the fact that not all campuses are created equal. This one can boast a multi-purpose gym, an aqua park

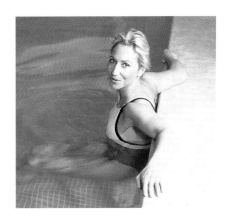

including an Olympic-sized pool, tennis courts, a 4km/2.5 mile cycling track around the campus and a chess room to get a brain workout as well as a brawn workout!
Praca 02, Prof. Rubiao Meira 61, Cidade Universitaria, Sao Paolo, Brazil
Tel: (+11) 3818 3565/3361

TOKYO

Club on the Park

If the price of membership does not give you a head rush, the altitude will. Located on the 47th floor of the Park Hyatt Hotel, this boasts a view of Mount Fuji on a clear day. When you are done with the myriad machines, equipment and workout gizmos, enjoy 360 body showers. And it really would be a shame to go all that way and not enjoy some ancient Oriental body treatments: reflexology or Shiatsu can be great to relieve that jet-lag.
Park Hyatt, 3-7-1-2 Nishi-Shinjuku – ku, Tokyo, Japan
Tel: (+81) 3 5322 1234

Workouts for free

Try some of these unforgettable jogging routes for an invigorating cardio blast.

DOMINICA

On the rainforest trail in Dominica's Northern Forest Reserve, through a parrot sanctuary, and up to the top of the island's highest mountain.

LONDON

Run east along the south bank of the Thames starting at Westminster Bridge and you will take in the famous sites – the Houses of Parliament, St Paul's Cathedral, the Tate Modern and Tower Bridge and back along the north embankment.

MINNEAPOLIS

Marvel at the beauty of the 'Chain of Lakes': the Lake of the Isles, Lake Calhoun and Lake Harriet.

PRAGUE

To take in the cultural views of Old Prague, start in Kampa park, run over Charles Bridge and then up to the impressive Castle. The hills can be pretty challenging as you stride past the wall that kept the poor out of the royal vista. Remember, power-walking can be great for your gluteals, so don't panic if you need to walk.

RIO DE JANEIRO

The route may be down hill but you need to be pretty fit to run all the way down to Copacabana beach. The running route through the national park is stunningly beautiful, so you may prefer to hire a mountain bike so that your enjoyment of the scenery is less arduous.

SYDNEY

Within walking distance of the city, Centennial Park offers a 4km/2.5 mile run against a car-free picturesque backdrop. Or if you fancy a more watery vista, start at Vaucluse and head along the coastal path down into Bondi, run along the beach and continue along the headlands and down into Tamarama. Running back to Vaucluse, you will be distracted on the last few hills, by the views of Sydney Harbour Bridge and the Opera House.

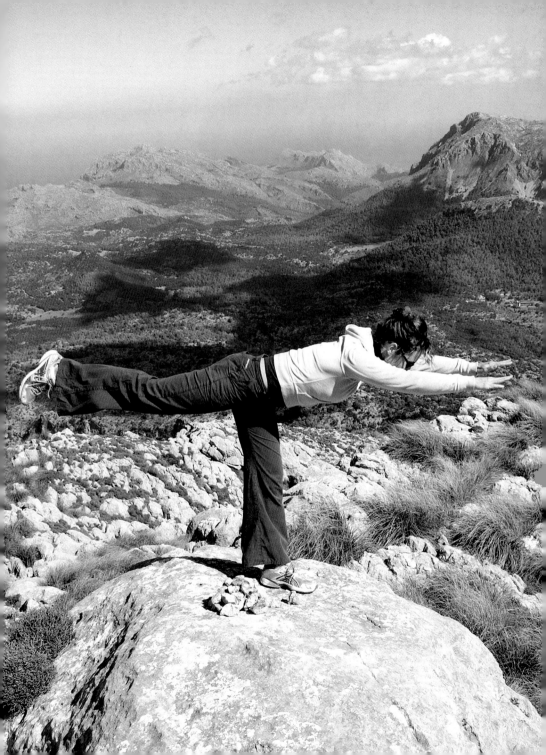

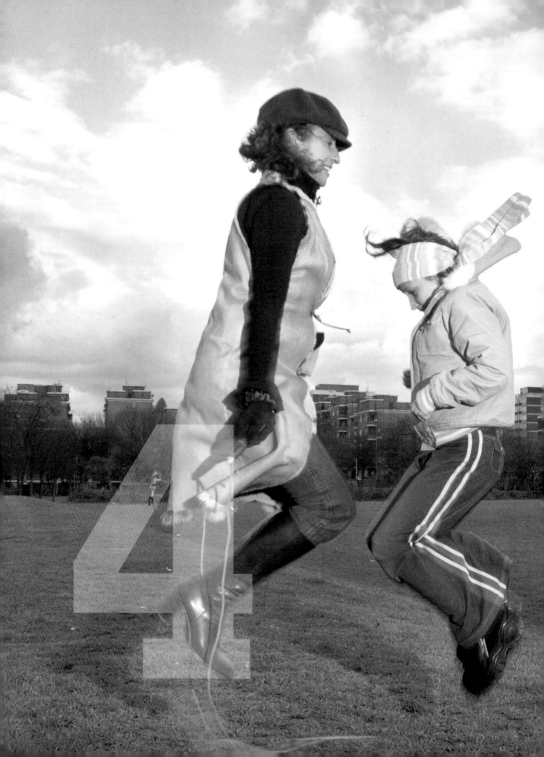

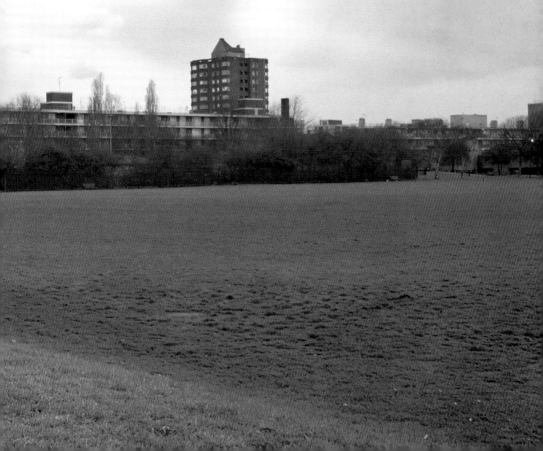

Your children's weight

Why are children gaining weight?

Children have always loved to jump, run and play; in fact, being active is the natural state of affairs for most kids. So how is it, then, that we are faced with a whole new generation of overweight children? Kids who choose the games console over playing in the park, watching TV over a bike ride with their friends, sitting slumped in front of a video rather than racing up and down the stairs? The food our children eat is obviously a major factor in their weight gain, but so too is this increased inactivity. It is a very simple equation; if they are inactive and eating the wrong foods, their weight will rise. And rise it has!

According to the International Obesity Task Force, some 22 million of the world's under-fives are now overweight or obese. In the UK, the government estimates that the number of overweight children has increased by 25 per cent since 1995, with almost 17 per cent of UK children now classified as obese. Obesity among six-year-olds has doubled in recent years to 8.5 per cent and trebled to 15 per cent among 15-year-olds – and note, these figures are for 'obese' children; not those who are simply overweight. Some leading medical experts warn that more than one in three adults, one in five boys and one in three girls will be obese by 2020 if current trends continue.

WON'T THEY OUTGROW IT?

The popular notion that most overweight children will 'lose their puppy fat' as they grow up is false. Baylor Medical School in the US reports that approximately 40 per cent of obese seven-year-olds and 70 per cent of obese adolescents become obese adults. The older your child gets, the harder it is for him to shift the weight, and the more likely it is he will be overweight or obese in adulthood.

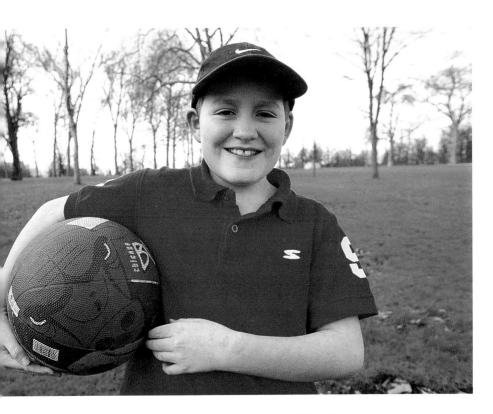

ASSESSING YOUR CHILD

Studies show that most parents simply do not consider their
children to be overweight, even when they are bordering on
obesity. Thankfully, the UK government has recognised this and
now supplies Body Mass Index charts in the health booklets
given to every child at birth (see page 30 for more about BMI).
Schools will also be helping parents keep tabs by monitoring
growth (height and weight) annually.

BMI AND CHILDREN

From the age of one you can plot your child's BMI on a standard
chart, which shows those of other children the same age.
Because what is normal changes with age (young children have
more 'baby fat', for instance), children's BMI measurements must
be plotted on paediatric BMI charts rather than assessed using

the normal range for adults. You use the same equation – weight in kilograms divided by height in metres squared – but on a different scale.

BMI declines from infancy to about five or six years of age, and then increases with age through childhood and adolescence. Kids tend to stick fairly closely to the same line throughout their childhood, and this is what you need to look at when working out if your child is obese: the real value of BMI measurements lies in viewing them as a pattern over time. For example, if your daughter shifts from the 50th to the 75th percentile, but remains there, she is probably growing in a way that is right for her. If you haven't kept a record of your child's weight and height across the years, you can start now.

NORMAL WEIGHT GAIN

It's also important to remember that many children do put on stores of fat in advance of a growth spurt, possibly during periods of illness, and always prior to and during adolescence. The distribution of weight also changes as children grow older. For example, from babyhood through to about five or six years of age, children accumulate more fat on their extremities than on their torsos. Then proportionally more fat accumulates around the tummy and trunk until adolescence. During the adolescent growth spurt, boys gain more fat on their trunks, while fat on their arms and legs decreases. Girls gain pretty much equal amounts of weight on their trunks, arms and legs during this period.

So the sudden appearance of a tummy after the age of six is not a sign of obesity, nor is this the case if your adolescent daughter suddenly develops more fat all over. It's worth remembering, too, that a child's body weight may double between the ages of 10 and 18.

DIFFERENT SHAPES AND SIZES

Some kids are whippet-thin and others sturdier and more muscular. A stocky child is not any more likely to be overweight than a child with the physique of a budding ballerina. Accept your child's body shape, but be on the look-out for signs that all is not well. For example, if you regularly buy clothes two or three

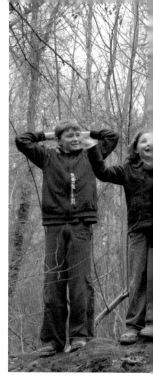

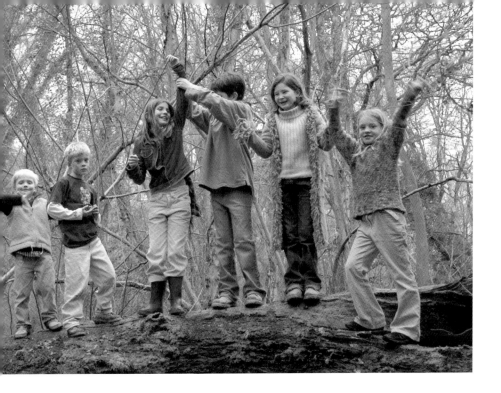

sizes larger than your child's age, or there are evident rolls of
fat or hefty deposits on his body, chances are he does have
weight problem.

GETTING THE BALANCE RIGHT

An overweight child is susceptible to some pretty serious health
problems, from diabetes and early heart disease to high blood
pressure, among other things. Overlooking the problem at an
early age can put your child in real danger of a lifetime of health
problems. So do you put your child on a diet?

Definitely not. Dieting is a definite no-no for children – not
only because it makes them feel 'different', but also because it
teaches them nothing about long-term healthy eating habits and
exercise – which are crucial to achieving balanced diets and
healthy weight. The key is to keep his weight stable so that he
'grows into' a healthy way of life. Healthy living is the goal rather
than watching the pounds fall off – but the wonderful byproduct
is that he slims down.

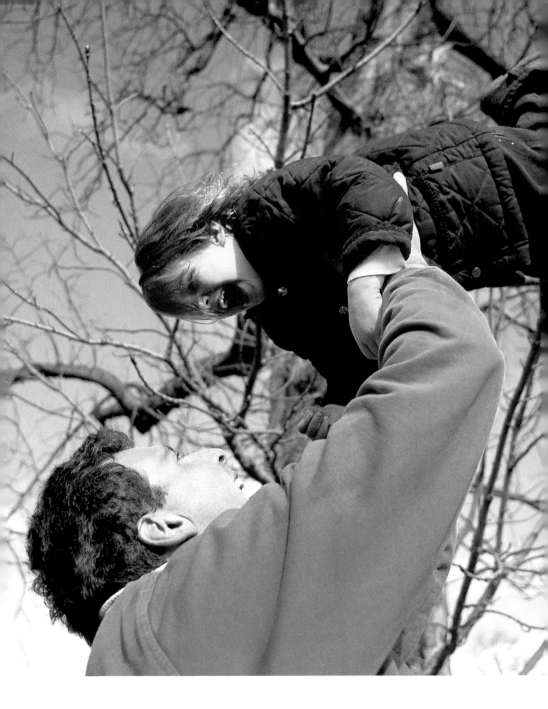

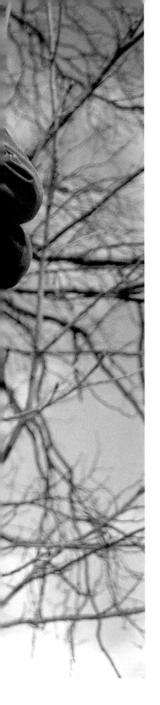

The importance of exercise

The best and only way to ensure that your child's weight stabilises is exercise – lots of it, and on a regular basis – complemented by a healthy diet. The key thing to remember, however, is that if the whole family is involved, your child will be much more likely to sustain his efforts.

A programme that involves just one family member will never work – they'll lose the motivation required to keep things going, and they'll be made to feel 'different'. Children learn by example and if everyone's doing it, good habits become a part of everyday life. Some say that ensuring that your child is more physically active instils a health benefit that is more powerful than medicine – and that's food for thought.

THE PARENTAL INFLUENCE

The body weight of a biological parent is the most reliable predictor of your child's body weight in adulthood – your child's chances of becoming an overweight adult are 80 per cent greater if either you or your partner is overweight. But genes play only a small part – most experts agree that it is your actions and behaviour that have the most influence. So make sure you set a good example.

HOW MUCH EXERCISE DO CHILDREN NEED?

The Chief Medical Officer recommends that children get a minimum of 60 minutes of at least moderate intensity physical exercise each day, plus activities designed to improve bone health, muscle strength and flexibility, at least twice a week. Currently 2 in 10 do less than 30 minutes of activity per day. Let's get planning how your children can meet the target.

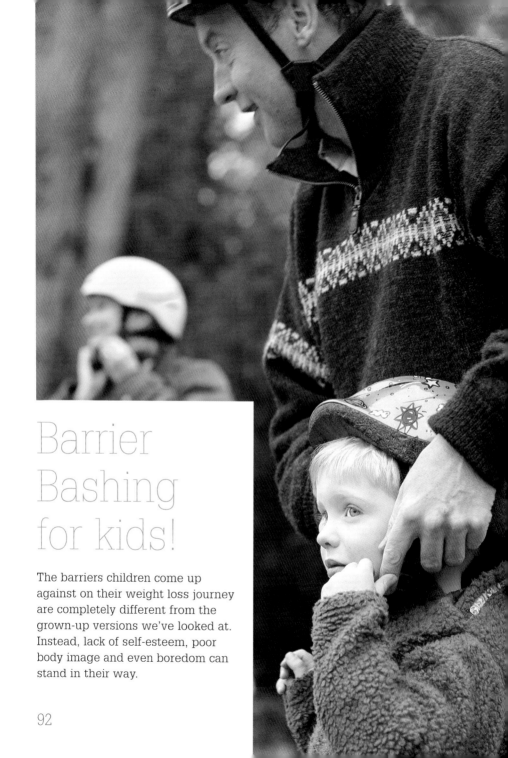

Barrier
Bashing
for kids!

The barriers children come up
against on their weight loss journey
are completely different from the
grown-up versions we've looked at.
Instead, lack of self-esteem, poor
body image and even boredom can
stand in their way.

FAMILY ACTIVITY TASK

Identify your and your child's personal barriers to physical activity. If you've worked your way through this book, you're probably well aware of your own by now, but nevertheless completing this task together with your child can be a useful exercise. Remember: as a parent you are leading by example. Draw up a list of your barriers and brainstorm possible solutions for dealing with each barrier in a form like the one on the right. Here's an example of a possible barrier:

BARRIER: LACK OF SELF-ESTEEM

Children may believe that they lack the skill required to exercise, or that their physical shape may hinder them. An obese child can feel uncomfortable about his body, and embarrassed about wearing exercise gear or swimming trunks. What's more, his size may make it harder for him to perform the activities required to expend energy.

Bash it down! Build in small victories, and nurture your child's Template of Success, as you do for yourself. But remember that while completing 120 seconds of activity 15 times a day may be a successful first step for you, for a child it will be meaningless – will-power is not a dominant characteristic in most kids, and they simply will not see the importance of doing something boring as a means to an end.

Children need to feel that they are good at something, so don't push them in the direction of a sport they dislike and for which they have little talent. Think more along the lines of games in the park, a basketball or football match with friends or other families, roller-blading or a ride on the scooter, or even badminton or 'beach volleyball' in the garden. This will get them playing hard or running fast for 30–60 seconds and resting for a minute or two before carrying on – essentially mimicking alternate brief bouts of vigorous exercise with longer recovery periods.

LEARNING TO LOVE TO MOVE

One of the most important aspects of your child's future health is helping them learn to love to move – it provides a powerful foundation to make physical activity and exercise part of adult life. Central to this will be making movement and exercise fun, and building their physical confidence so they experience success. Developing this at as early an age as you can is vital. Get those toddlers dancing!

FAMILY ACTIVITY TASK

To help your child learn to love to move, the first thing is to avoid competition: start with games that focus on participation and fun rather than skill.

- Enjoy early success: as skilled activities are introduced it is important that children experience early success, otherwise enthusiasm will quickly fade. A child's success ratio can be easily improved by creatively alternating various aspects of a game, and can be tailored to achieve success for children of different abilities and ages in the family. Younger members can have more goes and head starts; older players can help younger players.
- Ensure the environment is non-threatening: arrange activities in the garden or as a family in the local park, rather than taking them somewhere they may feel awkward and on display. Try to make activities group or family orientated, rather than showcases for personal success.
- Variety is the spice of life: take a traditional game or sport and modify it in an unusual way.

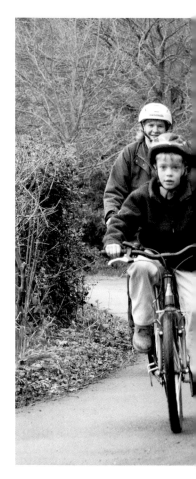

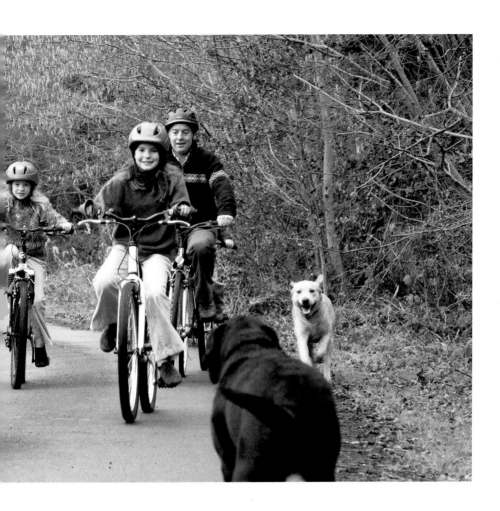

FIT FAMILY FACT: ON YOUR BIKE!

A young child is often less economical in her movements than an adult, but some modes of exercise can prove more effective for a child and hence build her self-confidence while she's still having fun. Cycling is one of the best all-round exercises a family can do together, because since it's independent of body weight and pedalling frequency (if the wheel size is the same), the mechanical efficiency of cycling is similar for children, adolescents and mums and dads! So plan a family cycling trip – why not bring a picnic and take a kite along?

HERE ARE SOME SUGGESTIONS:

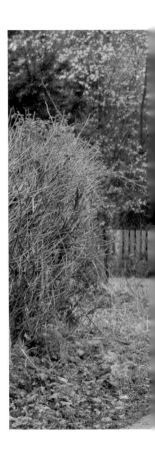

- Try 'beach cricket'– allow a player more than three goes, increase the size of the bat or ball, reduce the size of the field or run length, or try to hit off a stationary bowler. Alternate these variables to suit each player, thereby keeping the interest level up as well as increasing each child's success ratio.

- Set up an obstacle course in the garden, and time yourselves. Ask each family member to create an obstacle!

- Crab football is a great leveller! All the players sit down on the playing field and use their arms and legs to move about instead of running. The size of the pitch will need to be significantly smaller, but all other rules can remain the same. Altering activities like this not only improves overall motor co-ordination and control but also makes it much more interesting and much more fun. What's more, previous experience or talent is likely to be useless!

- Arrange a scavenger hunt, which can be an ideal game for a child to enjoy with an older relative, or in a larger group within your community. Start them off by making a list of items for the children and the older adults to look for on a walk, such as a bottle top, or a leaf or flower of a particular size or colour. At the end of the walk the group with the most items selects the next adventure or gets to write the next list of items to search for.

- 'History walks' with a grandchild and grandparent can be a great way for different generations to spend quality time together. Grandparents can shed some light on the past while both generations get some exercise.

- Initiate family walking projects. Give each member of the family a pedometer and ask them to log their steps on a family chart. A certain number of steps equates to a certain mileage and you can add them all up to reach a chosen destination. Making an older child responsible for the step chart helps give them a sense of fulfilment and keeps Mum and Dad on track with their walking too! Out of interest, add up the mileage to try to reach different countries. Get the atlas and the encyclopaedia out and use this opportunity to educate your children about different cultures. Or perhaps reward the whole family with a fun day out once the destination is reached.

- Make activity a normal part of life – wash the car together,

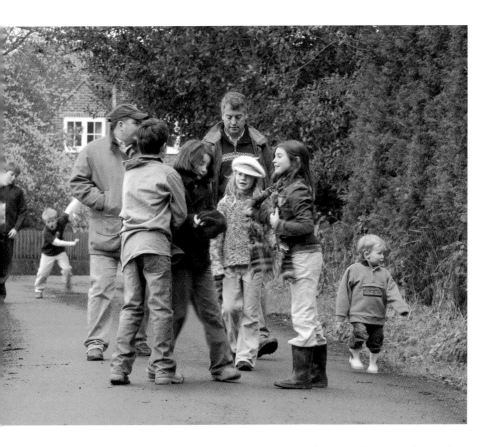

garden, mow the lawn, paint the house or the garden fence, clear
the junk in the garden shed – anything that gets kids and adults
up and out of the house. Give kids their own patch of garden to
plant what they like.

▪ Set up a net in the garden and play badminton, volleyball or
even 'tennis football' (keeping the ball in the air with feet and
heads only). If the weather is bad, most kitchen tables can be
easily turned into a table-tennis table.

▪ Have a sports day in the garden, complete with sack race,
three-legged race and egg and spoon race!

▪ Have a water fight with water balloons, a paddling pool, a
sprinkler and the garden hose. There's nothing that gets kids
and adults moving more quickly than a little cold water!

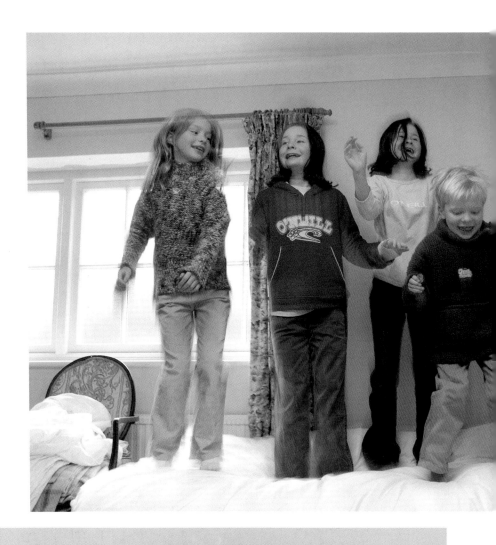

FIT FAMILY FACT: CHILDREN AND HEAT

Children have a much lower capacity to dissipate heat during exercise. A child's individual sweat glands form sweat more slowly and are less sensitive to increases in core body temperature than those of adults. Encourage your child to begin slowly and take several activity breaks and ensure they are wearing comfortable, loose-fitting clothing that will keep them cool and make them less conscious of their figure.

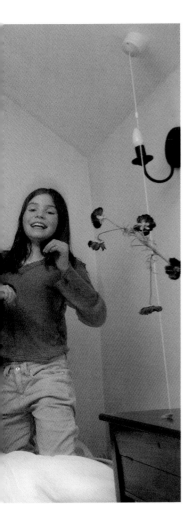

HELP KIDS TO BE SUCCESSFUL

If you want your children to stick to exercise, they need to feel good about themselves. Your child's first exercise experience is crucially important in shaping their attitude to exercise. Getting it right can be like knocking down the first domino – when the first one topples the rest will follow.

- Use positive reinforcement ('If you ride your bike, you can go to the cinema on Saturday'). Reacting to inactivity with the threat of punishment is a sure way to turn a child off exercise.
- Avoid saying anything potentially derogatory. It can be extremely painful to be overweight.
- Develop trust. Overweight kids are wary of exercise – so trust is a must. Don't ask your child to do anything you would not be prepared to do yourself.
- Understand children's bodies: be aware of the physical differences (see page 41–42) when you plan your activities.
- Empower kids: focus on getting children to be comfortable with who they are now and encourage them to become who they want to be.
- Reward every week where weight doesn't increase with a (non-food) token of progress – such as a trip to the cinema, a CD or a family outing. Try to avoid rewards that reinforce sedentary behaviours, such as Playstation games.
- Talk to your children about what is realistic, and don't promise miracles. Stress the benefits of healthier living, and point out that maintaining weight is an added benefit, rather than the sole reason for staying active and eating well.

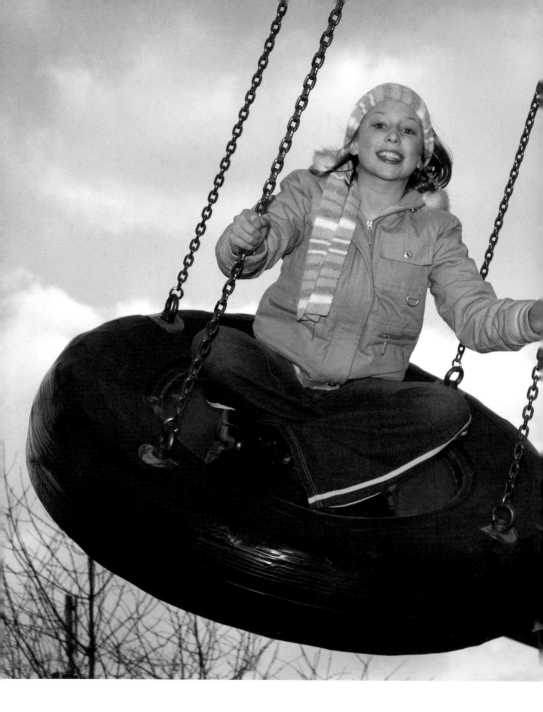

KEEP IT GOING!

Children will undoubtedly become more excited about active play if they have the right equipment. Balls, shinpads, bats, racquets, frisbees, basketball nets, swings and other outdoor toys or games make great birthday gifts or even 'rewards'. Make sure your children have what they need to play the games they want to play.

But encourage, too, a little imaginary play in the garden or the park – finding the shiniest conker, making snow or sand 'angels', building a fort, climbing a tree, 'catching' butterflies or falling leaves – anything that imbues them with a sense of fun and adventure in the outdoors. The pleasure they experience will turn them into adults who will choose a country walk over a beer in front of the telly!

FIT FAMILY FACT: HOW THEY MOVE

Children and adolescents are a lot less economical in their movements than adults, using more oxygen per body weight than adults do at any given walking or running speed. So if you choose to jog together, enter a fun run, or weekend rambling activity, it is very important that your child sets the pace. Remember to praise them for being active, rather than criticising them for being slow. This changes the older they get – younger members of the family should not be expected to keep up with their older siblings.

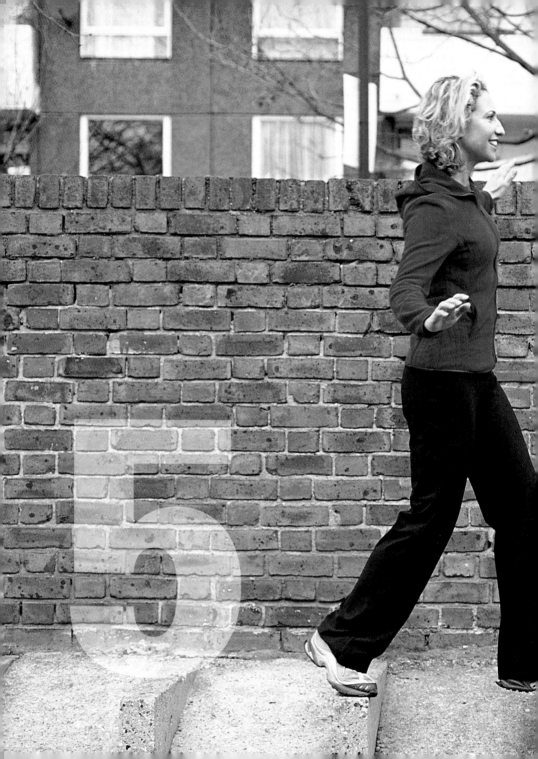

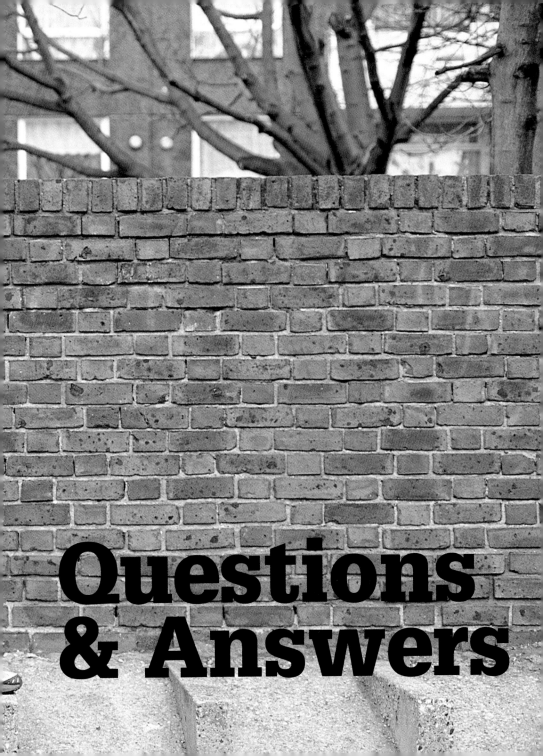

Questions
& Answers

"THE DIET I'M FOLLOWING IS VERY LOW CARB (JUST TWO SLICES OF WHOLE-GRAIN BREAD ALLOWED THREE TIMES A WEEK). I'VE LOST 17 POUNDS IN 7 WEEKS AND WOULD LIKE TO LOSE ANOTHER 30 POUNDS OVER THE NEXT 3 MONTHS, BUT DO I NEED MORE IN THE WAY OF CARBS?"

Congratulations on all of your hard work! Realistic and healthy goal setting is an important part of the weight loss process. If we set unrealistic goals, it can backfire and de-motivate us and re-inforce your Template of Failure – not what we want. A realistic and healthy weight loss goal is about 5 to 10 per cent of your current body weight in 3 to 6 months.

Watch the calories, not the carbs

It sounds as though your diet is focusing on healthy foods, but it would be a good idea to include some wholegrain starches every day, both for the fibre and for the B vitamins they provide. This shouldn't affect your rate of weight loss if you remember it is calories and not carbs that cause people to gain weight. Wholegrain cereal, crackers, pasta, bread, brown rice and low-fat popcorn are delicious and nutritious when eaten in moderation and operating my Carb Curfew is a useful way to keep your quantities in check.

"BECAUSE OF MY SHIFT I EAT LATE AT NIGHT WHEN I GET HOME. WHAT'S THE ABSOLUTE LATEST I SHOULD BE EATING, AND ARE THERE FOODS I SHOULD AVOID SO AS NOT TO TAX THE DIGESTIVE SYSTEM BEFORE I GO TO BED?"

Try to eat about one to two hours before you go to bed to allow your food to digest. Be sure to eat slowly and chew your food very well – digestion begins in the mouth, with the action of saliva.

Keep it simple

We are often tense or tired when we eat late at night, which can make us vulnerable to overeating. Use a small plate to remind yourself to eat smaller portions, and make sure that half of your plate is filled with colourful fruits and vegetables. Avoid spicy, fatty foods late at night, or those with rich, creamy sauces. Keep it simple – opt for soups and salads rather than an Indian takeaway.

"ACCORDING TO AN ONLINE CALORIE COUNTER, I SHOULD BE EATING BETWEEN 1,755 AND 2,025 CALORIES A DAY TO REACH MY GOAL. I'M ONLY EATING 1,400 BUT MY WEIGHT LOSS HAS STALLED. AM I EATING TOO LITTLE?"

Yes, that could be the case. When you're eating too few calories, your body gets a signal that you're starving, and all of your systems – your cardiovascular system, nervous system, gastrointestinal system, endocrine system – slow down, so that you're burning fewer calories and are better able to survive the 'famine'.

Count your calories carefully
I suggest that no one eats less than 1,500 calories a day except under medical supervision. But before you start eating more, make sure that you're counting everything you eat and drink accurately. If you're eating the right amount of calories and still not losing weight, see your doctor to check if you have metabolic problems.

"I THINK MY FRIEND MAY HAVE ANOREXIA. SHE HAS LOST A LOT OF WEIGHT RECENTLY AND SHE MAKES EXCUSES NOT TO EAT OUT WITH HER FRIENDS, SAYING SHE'LL JOIN US AFTERWARDS. WHAT SHOULD I DO?"

Anorexia nervosa is a disorder characterised by extreme weight loss and an intense fear of being fat. The disorder occurs most commonly in adolescent girls, but it is becoming more common in young men. People suffering from anorexia are very skinny and have often lost as much as a third of their body weight. They may exercise compulsively, and grow soft downy hair all over their body.

Get specialist help
If you suspect someone has an eating disorder such as anorexia or bulimia (a disorder in which sufferers binge eat and then induce vomiting), they need a lot of specialist support. Talk to your friend, but be prepared for denial and resistance. It may be helpful to contact the Eating Disorders Association (www.edauk.com, tel: 0845 634 1414); they will be able to give you advice on how to handle the situation.

"WHEN I FIRST STARTED EXERCISING I LOST WEIGHT QUICKLY. WHY CAN'T I DROP THE LAST FEW POUNDS?"

So you have lost the 'easy weight' – now comes the hard part! On any weight loss programme the greatest changes generally occur early on; and heavier, less fit people get more dramatic results at first. The closer you are to the last 2kg (5lb), the more effort you are going to have to put in.

Track your pulse

Trying a new activity can bring your resting pulse up, causing your body to burn more calories. Keep a tab on your resting pulse, as if it drops it could be a sign to shift your cardio training regime. Do some interval training at two sessions a week to trigger surges of growth hormone that promote fat burning. Maybe you should also do a reality check: the last 2kg (5lb) may be the hardest to lose because you are actually trying to get below your ideal weight.

"HELP! I'VE GOT CELLULITE! CAN I GET RID OF IT WITH DIET AND EXERCISE?"

Most experts agree cellulite is in part genetic, so the first thing I would suggest you do is take a look at the women in your family. However, your diet, exercise levels and body beauty routine can all affect the appearance of cellulite on your hips and thighs. Longer term, regular cardio exercise and decreasing the toxic load in your body by cutting back on processed foods and additives has been reported by some individuals to make a difference.

Get exercising

I suggest you introduce an interval cardio programme with 3-minute cardio bouts interspaced with compound large muscle group exercises. I would also suggest you try to minimise your alcohol and caffeine intake and cut right back on any artifical flavourings.

Body brushing

Some of my clients swear by rubbing a few drops of sweet fennel essential oil into their body moisturiser and rubbing in light upward sweeping movements on hips, thighs and bottom. You should also try dry body brushing before each shower. Sweep towards the groin lymph nodes to aid lymph drainage.

"I TRY TO EAT AS WELL AS I CAN, BUT RECENTLY I HAVE BEEN BINGEING ON JUNK FOOD LATE AT NIGHT FOR NO REASON. I EXERCISE REGULARLY AND EAT WELL THE REST OF THE TIME. HOW CAN I STOP MYSELF BINGEING?"

It seems on the surface that you are doing the right things in your diet and exercise, but you are not in the right head space! Although you are exercising, your brain seems to expect you to fail and let yourself down. Have you followed a lot of different diets in the past, especially extreme quick-fix ones? In my experience, this can cause low self-esteem; you start to doubt that your actions will work.

Build a Template of Success

To do this I suggest you pick three small things that can be building blocks each week to help you towards your goal. For example, operate my Carb Curfew after 5pm; just say no to bread, pasta, rice and potatoes and instead focus your evening meal on lean meat, fish, fruit and veg with some essential fats. This will help you to cut down your calorie intake and will also reduce bloating. On top of this, be sure to drink your 2 litres of water a day, and take a brisk 10-minute walk before you sit down at your desk. All these small actions add up and help you build a Template of Success! Look at the 7 Steps to Self Esteem on pages 12–15 to help analyse your attitude further.

keep yourself thin

107

"I DO LOADS OF SIT-UPS BUT I STILL HAVE A JELLY BELLY – WHAT AM I DOING WRONG?"

Sit-ups are technically a toning exercise designed to challenge the abdominal group of muscles. Performing sit-ups with good technique will help to tighten, flatten and strengthen your abdominals. However these muscles lie under a layer of adipose (fat) tissue. If you are not over-eating, the excess abdominal fat may be a sign of too much tension and stress. Long-term chronic stress that goes unchecked creates a build-up of the stress hormone cortisol. Cortisol creates a challenge to weight loss on two levels: first it increases appetite, especially the urge for sugary sweets, and second it encourages these excess calories to be laid down around the midriff area.

Add sweat to your sit-ups

Any vigorous exercise helps reduce overall body fat, including that tummy. While it was once thought we were born with a certain number of fat cells, scientists now believe that once our existing fat cells reach a critical size they split, creating more fat cells. To keep the fat off your midriff you need to make cardio exercise a regular feature of your training programme.

Control your stress

Try to build a stress reducer into your daily life – this will be different for each of us, but yoga, listening to relaxing music, enjoying a soothing bath and walking can be great stress reducers, which will help regulate your cortisol levels and keep that belly bulge at bay. Getting enough good quality sleep is important too; studies have shown getting 6 versus 8 hours of sleep increases cortisol output by 40 per cent.

Ban the booze

Alcohol is very calorie dense. Every gram contains 7 calories, almost twice as much as protein and carbohydrates. In addition research shows that some types of alcohol – mainly beer – can cause more fat to settle on your belly.

"MY FRIEND AND I EAT AND EXERCISE THE SAME, YET SHE'S ONLY THE ONE LOSING WEIGHT. WHY HER AND NOT ME? IT'S JUST NOT FAIR."

To get the answer to this one, you need to look at your parents. If you had an overweight parent then you have a 79 per cent greater chance of having weight problems as an adult. (Your chances are slightly higher if it was your Mum.) Genetics affect our shape and how our bodies respond to food and exercise by as much as 40 per cent. But before you toss in the towel remember that your DNA is not your destiny. The most effective change you can make is to become a regular exerciser and make it a consistent five-times-a-week habit. If you burn an extra 30 calories an hour during the 14 to 16 hours that you are awake – by taking the stairs or walking briskly instead of dawdling – you could incinerate up to 500 extra calories a day without doing an actual workout. You could even overtake your friend!

Remember that as you set out on your weight-loss journey, it's important to be realistic about what you can achieve. There may never be a 'perfect time' for you to begin your action plan, so don't wait for the perfect time – in my experience, if you adopt this attitude you'll never get past the starting line.

Your long-term success will depend upon how well you navigate your time from now on, and how you choose to live your life. If you have the desire to lose weight and are willing to put in some effort, you will succeed. Remember that each small step you take along the way will make a big difference. You can do this! Go for it!

Resources

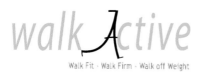

Walkactive - Joanna's Online Walking Club

Joanna's company, Walkactive, is a company committed to helping people make walking work for them. Walkactive offers a range of walking events, trainer-led courses, Walking Spa breaks, online programmes, support club and products all designed by Joanna so that you can Walk Fit, Walk Firm and Walk Off Weight.

On our Walk Off Weight and Walk Fit programmes our clients typically benefit from:

- up to a 10-inch loss in body shape
- up to 10 pounds in weight loss
- a 25% increase in cardiovascular fitness in just 6 weeks

Becoming a member of Joanna's Walkactive online club gives you a whole host of benefits...

Club benefits include:
- A Joanna Hall Steps pedometer (worth £15)
- Our certified 100% organic 'Walkactive' T-shirt (worth £15.99)

- Discounts and priority booking on all Walkactive walking courses, walking spa breaks, walking workshops and events with Joanna
- Get real body results – exclusive downloadable walking programmes personally designed by Joanna – so you know they work!
- Keep motivated – with weekly e-mail support and motivation, daily-step log charts and weekly tracking progress charts
- Stay on track with Joanna's personal advice and online chats
- Meet fellow walkers and exchange tips on our online forums
- Access to Charity walking event listings with member ratings and reviews on Charity events and products
- Save money on all 'Walkactive' and Joanna Hall books, dvds and pedometers and get amazing discounts at specialist retailers and outlets

To join and for more information, go to:
www.walkactive.co.uk

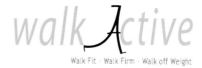

Walkactive is a registered trademark of Joanna Hall Lifestyle Management

WHERE TO SHOP

Cassall
Stylish active wear clothing available online at www.sportswoman.co.uk and in store at John Lewis

Joanna Hall pedometers, books and exercise DVDs
www.joannahall.com

Joanna's Walk Fit, Walk Firm, Walk Off weight events, courses and spa breaks
www.walkactive.co.uk

Juicers
www.ukjuicers.com

Menopause matters
an independent, clinician-led website that provides accurate information about the menopause
www.menopausematters.co.uk

Sweaty Betty for exercise clothing
www.sweatybetty.com

She Active for exercise clothing
www.sheactive.co.uk

Shoes
Healthy walking shoes for work and leisure
www.lovethoseshoes.com

Tanita Body Fat Scales and Skipping Ropes
www.tanita.com

GENERAL HEALTH

British Nutrition Foundation
For information about healthy eating and weight loss:
www.nutrition.org.uk (tel. 020 7404 6504)

British Heart Foundation
For details of 30 a day and other campaigns: www.bhf.org.uk
(tel. 020 7935 0185)

Chartered Society of Physiotherapy
For advice and tips on healthy posture:
csp.org.uk (tel. 020 7306 6666)

National Osteoporosis Society
nos.org.uk (tel. 0845 130 3076) for information about how exercise can build strong bones

Index

Achievements,
    acknowledging, 14
Action plans, 48–51
Alcohol, 67
Anorexia nervosa, 105

Barriers to weight loss
    arriving home starving, 66
    bashing, 22–25, 66–79
    binge-eating, 76, 77
    buffets, 75
    chocolate hour, 68
    effort required, 23
    evening crisp craving, 68
    going out to dinner, 70–73
    hunger after dinner, 69
    ice-cream urge, 69
    kids, for, 92–101
    knowledge, lack of, 24
    obstacles, 25
    party time, 66, 67
    proper dinner, no time for,
        74
    self-esteem, lack of, 24
    stress cravings, 68
    support, lack of, 23, 24
    time, lack of, 23
    travelling, 77–79
    weekends, 76
Body composition,
    measuring, 29–35
Body fat percentage, 33
Body frame, 38
Body, life journey, 40–47
Body mass index, 31
Body measurement, 29–35
Body shapes, 36–39
Bravery, revisiting acts of, 14

Calcium deficiency, 52
Carb curfew, 63
Cellulite, 106

Children
    barrier bashing, 92–101
    exercise, 41, 91
    heart rates, 41
    self-esteem, lack of, 93
    teens, in, 42
    weight, gaining, 86–89

Eating out, 70–73
Eyestrain buster, 62

Forgiving yourself, 15

G-spot motivation, 18, 19
Genes, 52, 109
Girth measurement, 34, 35
Goal-setting, 20, 21
Gym locations, 80, 81

Hormones,
    effect on shape, 39
Hunger drive, 52

Insulin resistance, 53

Late, eating, 104
Lemon drink, wake-up, 60
Liquid calories, 67
Low-carb diet, 104

Meditation, 65
Menopause, 47
Middle-age spread, 50
Modern living, effect, 52

Naked, getting, 17
Negativity, getting rid of, 13

Occupational lifestyle, 79

Parties, 66, 67
Past situations,

dealing with, 15
Pedestal,
    putting yourself on, 16, 17
Peri-menopause, 46
Portion distortion, 64
Pregnancy,
    weight gain in, 44

Seasonal Affective Disorder,
    54
Self-esteem, 12–15, 24
    children, 93
Sit-ups, 108
Sleep exercise, 65
Smoking, 49
Stress
    cravings, 68
    effect on weight, 55
    hormones, 53
Success
    listing, 14
    measuring, 25
    template of, 11
Systematic relaxation, 65

T'ai chi, 51
Time, making, 16, 23
Travelling, 77–79

Waist circumference, 32
Waist-to-hip ratio, 32
Weight, change in, 10
Weight loss
    barrier-bashing, 22–25,
        66–79
    day, navigating, 58–65
    factors affecting, 52–55
    goals, 20, 21
    maintaining, 58–65
    stalling, 105
    success, measuring, 25
Workouts, free, 82